T0153229

LEARNING TO LOVE
THE SPACES IN BETWEEN

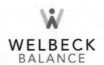

WELBECK
BALANCE

LEARNING TO LOVE
THE SPACES IN BETWEEN

Discover the Power of Liminal Spaces

By Claire Gillman

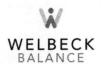

WELBECK
BALANCE

Published in 2022 by Welbeck Balance
An imprint of Welbeck Trigger Ltd
Part of Welbeck Publishing Group
Based in London and Sydney
www.welbeckpublishing.com

Design and layout © Welbeck Trigger Ltd 2022
Text © Claire Gillman 2022

A CIP catalogue record for this book is available from the British Library.

ISBN
Trade Paperback – 978-1-80129-114-9

Typeset by Lapiz Digital Services
Printed in Great Britain by CPI Group (UK) Ltd, Croydon CRO 4YY

10 9 8 7 6 5 4 3 2 1

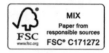

MIX
Paper from
responsible sources
FSC® C171272

To my wonderful and much missed mum, Pat Gillman
(15.6.1921 – 24.10.2020)

CONTENTS

INTRODUCTION TO LIMINALITY – AND MY FASCINATION WITH IT

Back in my early twenties, as a young journalist I had the good fortune to be sent on a press trip to cover a walking holiday in the wilds of the Scottish Highlands. Each day, the guide would take us to a different glen or hill, and while he accompanied the older, less fit journalist on the trip, I was allowed to ramble ahead among the gorse and heather on my own. It was on that trip, as the cloud hung low above the vast and empty purplish hillsides, that I first experienced a spine-tingling sensation of heightened sensory awareness and strong feeling of otherworldliness. The landscape itself was mystical and full of an indescribable energy. I felt as though I was on the edge of something inexplicably numinous, physical yet metaphysical at the same time. I was aware of something greater than myself. In the evening, in front of a blazing fire, I tried to explain my odd experience to the guide, hoping that I wouldn't sound entirely mad. As a local, he didn't bat an eyelid and told me that I was in a 'thin place', experiencing the liminal. That was the first time I had heard the expression, liminal space. Ever since,

I have been drawn to those locations and to that awe-inspiring feeling. Liminality fascinates me.

The word 'liminal' comes from the Latin 'līmen', meaning 'threshold.' In its literal sense, a threshold is a doorway. Liminal is often used to describe the threshold, or gateway, between two stages. Its contemporary definition in the Marriam-Webster dictionary is either 'of or situated at a sensory threshold – barely perceptible' or 'relating to or being in an intermediate state, phase or condition – transitional'. In anthropology, it is used to describe the ambiguity or disorientation that occurs in the middle phase of a rite of passage, while in psychology it defines the process of transitioning across boundaries or borders. Architecture sees it as the physical spaces between one destination and the next, such as hallways, tunnels, airports, carparks and corridors. Impermanence, transition, intermediary and threshold are the themes that link these multiple meanings.

As the years passed, my interest in the liminal grew, but when pressed, I found it hard to explain what it was about the subject that drew me. To be more accurate, I found it hard to even explain what liminality was. I would start by saying that liminality is 'the spaces and times inbetween' – the transitional moments and mystical places that we experience in our lives. As examples, I would talk about physical geographical spots, such as the coastline – where the land meets the sea – a perfect and readily understandable example of liminal space, and coincidentally a place where I love to spend time and to which many of us are drawn. I'd also talk of spiritual 'thin places' where 'heaven and earth feel closer', as first experienced on that trip to the Highlands.

When I tried to describe liminality further by launching into a description of the metaphysical space that is consciousness or the hypnagogic liminal state between sleep and wakefulness, I'd see people's eyes start to glaze over like marbles and so I realized that I needed to explore the notion of liminality further, in order to be able to fully explain it.

What to Expect

Given our recent unnerving experiences of liminality during the uncertainty of the pandemic, it seemed pertinent to start our journey of exploration with a look at the effects of the unbidden periods of change that inevitably occur in our lives in **Chapter 1: Transition and Change – the Fertile Void**. How can we best navigate these turbulent periods in our lives and optimize the pause in perspective that they offer?

Of course, the one unavoidable transition for everyone is the liminality of life. **Chapter 2: Hovering Between Life and Death** looks at the transition as we pass from this life, and also delves into the views and research of those who have studied Near Death Experiences (NDEs) and Out of Body Experiences (OBEs).

Reports from experiencers of NDEs and OBEs, particularly when they were medically and clinically considered dead, led me to question the liminality of consciousness itself and whether it can indeed be sited in the brain? This topic, which so divides the scientific and medical world, forms **Chapter 3: Opening the Doors of Perception**.

Since it transpires that many people voluntarily seek to explore liminality and all that it can offer within an altered consciousness, **Chapter 4: Mind-Altering Practices and Substances** looks into the role of mind-altering substances, both natural and man-made, such as magic mushrooms, ayahuasca, ketamine and LSD, and higher-consciousness practices such as chanting, drumming and meditation.

This naturally leads on to **Chapter 5: Tapping Into the Divine** and the liminality of spirituality, divinity and prayer. Who or what are we connecting to when we communicate with a higher power or the Divine?

From here, our odyssey of investigation expands its scope from the metaphysical to the physical, as we look into the power and attraction of the liminal times in the day, the seasonal calendar and nature's cycles in **Chapter 6: Tuning In to Natural Phases and Cycles**. Understanding more about being in tune with nature only served to pique my curiosity further about those places in our landscape that we are most drawn to – the wild places on the edge, the 'thin places', the sacred sites and the purpose of pilgrimage to such places – **Chapter 7: Wilderness, Thin Places and Pilgrimage**.

Finally, the search for answers about liminality led me to the global stage, with an exploration of how humanity finds itself teetering on the brink of ecological disaster in **Chapter 8: Our Natural World on the Brink**.

You can see just how vast and broad the topic of liminality is. You might be drawn to one aspect of it, say, the metaphysical rather than the geophysical, or the other way around. At the end of each chapter, I set out the take-aways that I have gleaned from those willing and generous experts who shared their wisdom, plus practical suggestions from myself and the experts that you might want to incorporate into your life view, to better understand and embrace the power of liminal spaces.

The Writing Process

The old saying goes, 'If you want to give the gods a laugh, tell them your plans.' In March 2020, the world was rocked by the global COVID pandemic, and this book project was promptly shelved. With our health under threat, lifestyles curtailed and indelibly altered, and our futures unclear, we found ourselves living in uncertain times. Few of us were immune from the unsettling feeling of being in transition.

Bizarrely though, for me, while lamenting the suffering and loss of life caused by the virus, I could also see how the feelings of being in limbo and on the brink of something unknown caused by the pandemic had given each of us a clearer understanding of liminality – the spaces and times where the known ceases to exist, where transformation takes place, the place in between the familiar and the unfamiliar.

Suddenly, when I used the example of the effects of lockdowns and COVID on the global population as a way to explain liminality, my enquirers had their own personal glimpse and thus a better understanding of what I was talking about. However, I felt the pandemic served only to show people how unnerving liminal space can be, how discombobulating and disconcerting. How downright terrifying. Instinctively, I felt that liminality, in all its guises, could also be a place where insight, creativity and inspiration are found. By accepting liminality into our lives, it has the potential to produce a sense of awe in us. In an age where so much is known, defined and explained, the feelings we derive from liminal spaces and times can shake up our complacency and enchant us if we let them.

As the pandemic restrictions eased, I started to compile my list of the aspects of liminality I needed to explore, reaching out to experts within those fields. Having spent almost 20 years as a contributor and/or editor for *Kindred Spirit* magazine, the UK's leading guide to conscious living and wellbeing, I was exposed to countless different modalities, esoteric subjects, and both traditional and cutting-edge teachings. I was also lucky enough to have interviewed amazing and inspiring thought-leaders committed to helping others and making the world a better place to live. Some of these luminaries were the first people that I approached.

To my surprise and utter delight, most of these highly respected experts were only too happy to share their knowledge, wisdom and enthusiasm for their subject. At the outset, however, I didn't quite understand how much of a double-edged sword all this insightful information would turn out to be. The deeper I dived into liminality, the more rabbit holes I ran down. The more answers I was given, the more questions were prompted in me. Little had I suspected that in the researching and writing of this book, the process would turn into my very own experience of being in the unknown, lost in the choppy waters of uncertainty.

I am far from inexperienced in the process of writing books, yet the writing process for this book was unlike any that I had experienced before. In the middle of the project, I found myself somewhat adrift, unsure of how best to pull together all that I was learning. The concept for the book changed and evolved.

And just as I had intuitively suspected at the outset, from the deeply uncomfortable and, for me, unusual place of not knowing how this book could best work, from that liminal space, a lightbulb moment emerged; this book became a documentary of my own investigation into liminal spaces, and I hope you find the voyage as engaging as I did.

I came to understand how liminality is all around us in our daily lives, how it affects our decision-making and our creativity; how exploring it can help us to better understand ourselves and our place in the Universe; and why welcoming change and liminality into our lives, rather than actively avoiding it, can be a good thing for us all. I'm left in no doubt that to more fully know ourselves and to be in harmony with the world around us, we need to lose ourselves in liminal space whenever possible.

1

TRANSITION AND CHANGE - THE FERTILE VOID

Each and every one of us had a taste of being in the liminal during the COVID pandemic, where our trusted and true way of life was turned on its head and the shape of our future on the other side seemed uncertain.

In the midst of this confusing and challenging period, I saw an article in the July 2021 issue of *Elle* magazine entitled 'Inbetweeners', and a pull-out quote jumped out at me. It read: "What if setbacks were a rite of passage toward a new version of ourselves?" After reading the article, I tracked down the author, Abigail Bergstrom, an author and publisher, to ask her about the dramatic life choices she made in the midst of a global pandemic.

Bergstrom had experienced a kind of burnout at work and, after a period of sick leave, she says, "I knew I needed to do something drastic." So she quit her job.

"I was jobless, which is the most insane thing for me, because my identity is so closely knitted in with what I do for a living. My job was everything. It's what I care about, it's my purpose, why I get out of bed in the mornings, what drives conversations with new people that I meet.

And, while that's great and a privilege, it can also be incredibly toxic when all of your value and all of your worth is inextricably linked to how you're showing up in your career. For me, that balance was way off. So, I literally severed that connection, was unemployed there and then, and had no conception of what I was going to do."

At the same time she left a very successful job in publishing, Bergstrom also gave up her home due to the pandemic to move in with her boyfriend, which in itself was a young relationship, to start over again in a new location.

Why had she chosen to embrace the uncertainty of a liminal life? I asked her. "The fact that the pandemic was at its crisis point weirdly spurred me on," she replied. "It maybe made it seem more acceptable that you could make your life a bit more chaotic and in flux, subject to change and that unknowability as well. I'd been living in my flat with my dog, single, independent, and then I met Mark. We were very much trapped in that liminal space in the sense that we moved into a house, but of course, it was a temporary solution. My permanent solution – my flat, my home – I'd let go of. Being separated from my own stuff, those key identifiers – the books we own, the objects we carry around with us or the blankets that we love that our grandmothers knitted for us, whatever it is that mirrors back who we are – and living without them was strange and frightening."

Knowing how disconcerting I had found the uncertainty of the pandemic, I asked her how it felt to find herself suddenly in this liminal space? Her candid reply: "It was terrifying. But it was also amazing, because for the first time ever, my key identifiers, like how people see me from the outside world or even how I see myself, weren't there. They didn't exist. I had somewhere to live but I was homeless in the sense of having my own curated home. Similarly with the job. It was almost like I had no idea who I was anymore. While that's horrible, it also created space for me to put different hats on and to think, 'Maybe I just want to go and work in a bookshop and have a quieter life?' or 'Perhaps I could live in Portugal?'"

As Abigail Bergstrom was finding out, liminality provides fertile ground for creative exploration of self. When your world is fixed and rigid, it can be hard to shake things up and explore other possible versions of yourself. By throwing her life up in the air, Bergstrom had the perfect opportunity to try out different options. It was the first time in her adult professional life that she wasn't subject to regimented time constraints. "That was the biggest thing that I learned about myself, that I was living in a way where every single moment of my time was apportioned: 7am – wake up, 20 minutes to shower, 10 minutes to put on make-up and make a cup of coffee, 10 minutes to take the dog for a walk. Leave the house and call client on the way to the Tube; get off the Tube and 10 minutes later, have your first meeting; get out of meeting, go to the next meeting. It was insane. I would run from the office to have my bikini wax, and I'd be catching up on emails while there, then I'd run back to my office for the next meeting. In the evening I would go to a work event and then try to catch up with friends for drinks and the dinners I had missed. I couldn't see at the time but there was no let up. I got to the point where I was siphoning off my weekends to rest in order to be able to keep up with the job, which is an awful way to live.

"For me, the biggest thing that I learned was that I cannot continue to have that relationship with time. I need to be more fluid. I can't live in this stringent, anxiety-induced place where I'm obsessively letting time rule my life and document my day. So that was the thing liminal space showed me."

The Fertile Void

I wondered whether Abigail Bergstrom would have had these self-realizations and insights into what was working in her life and what was not if she hadn't taken such a radical leap of faith into this liminal space and left her old life behind completely? Could this greater understanding have come to her without such a drastic upheaval? There is no hesitation in her response. She says, "It was absolutely necessary. For me, the liminal space gave me the chance to sit with and really look at the way that I was living. The only way I could have grasped that fully was to have stopped living that way.

"In a way, it was complete and utter heaven. That's the weird thing about liminal spaces; they're like your worst nightmare, but absolute bliss. In a way, it's almost like coming back to yourself, because you're less preoccupied with the external moments in time, or those external key identifying pillars."

Bergstrom returned to work in 2021 and set up Bergstrom Studio, a publishing consultancy and agency. Now that she had consciously let go of the safety of shore and launched into the uncertainty of the liminal seas, I asked Bergstrom if she discovered any other profound possibilities that exist within this "fertile void", as she described it in the article? "I feel less afraid of not having those things that I think society teaches us we must have; we must have these things sorted out for ourselves and organized into neat little boxes that other people understand and can reference. Being in liminality has made me feel less fearful about what happens in life. I feel more independent. It made me feel fortified. It was never an ambition of mine to set up my own agency, and yet, falling into that liminality, being in a different space, instinctively, it just felt like the next step. Maybe I didn't think that I had what it took to set up my own business and being in this liminal space showed me that I was capable. It made me have that self-belief."

This statement felt to me as though the very act of taking a leap of faith into the unknown and coming safely out the other side (not a given I suppose) both more resilient and more self-reliant was akin to a rite of passage. Did Bergstrom think of it in the same terms? "You can suspect how you would react or how you might cope, but until you've done it, you don't really know that about yourself. You think that you might be somebody who wouldn't cope with liminality at all, and that it would be your worst nightmare. And yet, it can happen and you could love it. I loved it. Looking at yourself in a really intense way and taking away those distractions that we create for ourselves to make us feel safe is uncomfortable, but you can't answer those questions unless you've been to that place of chaos and uncertainty."

Finding a Catalyst

In truth, uncertainty is a state that causes, at the very least, anxiety in most of us, and fear in others. Not just the fear of liminality in and of itself, but fear that we don't have the emotional resources to cope with the unknown quality of this state. Of course, unexpected transitions and changes are going to be sprung upon us at some point in our lives, but it is rare that someone actively chooses to let go of all that is familiar without something else in place, as Abigail Bergstrom did.

Psychologically and emotionally we crave homeostasis and predictability, though there are times in our lives when a decision or change is necessary and we're just not sure what to do or are uneasy about making the wrong decision. At times like these, talking about your dilemma or taking yourself off to get a different perspective on your life can be helpful. I have attended a course that helps you to find the space to do this and know the founder John Parkin well. I first wrote about the 'F**k It' retreats he runs with his wife in Italy back in 2008, and can testify to the transformational effects many attendees report. I spoke to Parkin about the philosophy behind his course and his books, the first of which, *F**k It: The ultimate spiritual way*, has just been updated and rereleased.

He explained: "With the profanity of F**k It, it's allowed people the courage to get out of the rut and off the path into something less certain. The main point really of the classic F**k It teaching is that instead of doing what we think we should do or what we've been told we ought to do or achieve, we should be more in tune with what's going on inside us."

Parkin himself has personal experience of turning his back on convention. In their early thirties, he and his wife Gaia Pollini left their well-paid jobs in an advertising agency in London and, together with their infant twin sons, headed off to a remote part of Le Marche, a region in northern Italy, to open a retreat called The Hill That Breathes. There, they taught their F**k It retreats on the art of giving less of a damn. Where did this irreverent, unconventional approach come from, I wondered?

Parkin says, "I think some of the trusting and leaping has been a reaction to my upbringing. My parents are very phobic of change or risk. I have a backdrop of 'everything needs to be controlled and predicted, set up and planned.' So, it was liberating for me to strike out and to go and do things differently, but not just in that kind of teenage way of reacting. There was no real ability in my family to be in discomfort or in conflict. No ability to be in the uncertainty, so I have really welcomed in my life the chance to be in the question, in the discomfort of things. That space you're talking about, the liminal space, it seems to me that it is a necessary space if you're moving from one zone of certainty to another. You have to be okay to be in the question before the question is answered. I've realized that the 'corridors' of my life, the times when I didn't know quite which door would open, have been the most interesting, and I'm wondering if the gentle tension of those times was critical to that interestingness."

Desire for Certainty

Despite our default desire for certainty and security, there will always be unavoidable transitionary periods in our lives, which can be thought of as liminal space. Whether it's divorce or illness, grief or graduation, moving location or job change, some life phases will be longer than others, and some will be harder than others but, of course, liminality always has an endpoint. The trick is becoming more comfortable during the transition process itself.

Despite uprooting their life several times, John Parkin surprises me by telling me that he too has a powerful natural desire for safety – but he has come to realize that the reality of life is that it's always moving around and changing. He says, "I'm aware that in my psyche is a great desire for certainty but whenever I get close, some part of it slips away, which, for me, is life telling me that this is how it will always be. So, the invitation that I've always had is how can I be in the bit where I don't need security and certainty? How can I be okay in this space? I try to focus on the fact that things always tend to work out and the more relaxed I am about the uncertainty, the better it seems to work out. The more I allow the situation to move, the more it seems to be okay.

"On the F**k It weeks, we would talk about how we live in this frozen mid-land of life where we won't really go for it, because we're so scared of what can go wrong. We never go either side of this frozen mid place. Yet when you relax and let everything melt, it's like all the emotions start to come up, and all the opportunities come up, and you begin to do things that you wouldn't normally do. The liminal is where there's more movement. It's where the ice melts, where you have to be open to things going wrong, and the uncertainty of it and the potential pain and the mess of it, and then, great things come as well, because that's what happens when it melts and it moves."

Creativity in the Liminal

These words rang true to me in relation to the creative process that went into the writing of this book, probably more so than any of my previous books. I can honestly say that the concept that I started with changed, melted and morphed into something completely different by the end, but in the midst of that process, I found myself at a loss as to how this book would come to fruition, if at all. How could I translate my thoughts and the wonderful wisdom of all the interviewees into something cohesive and accessible for a wider audience? It became a creative liminal process in which I lost my original idea of what the book was going to be, sat in the discomfort of not knowing, and came out the other side with a different version. I must confess, it was a disquieting experience until the creative answer eventually came clear, and then it felt amazing.

Psychotherapist, broadcaster and author Robert Holden specialises in positive psychology and wellbeing, and hosts the weekly radio show *Shift Happens!* As the author of over a dozen books, his latest being *Higher Purpose*, I asked him about his creative process. He says, "One of the things about the liminal space, especially with writing and with creativity, is that you have to let yourself be lost if you are going to be guided. Most of us don't like to feel lost. We are taught to be definite about where we are going, even if it's the wrong direction. Lost sounds like we're admitting to a failure, but actually, we have to be able to say in the creative process, and in the healing journey, 'I'm completely lost and I'm willing to be guided. I'm completely lost and I'm going to let myself be more open than before, more available than before. I'm going to be uncertain in this moment, so that I can receive some sort of guidance.'

"I find in the creative process, in particular writing a book, you meet the blank page over and over again. You sit there and you go, 'Maybe this book was never meant to be. Okay, I'm lost. I don't know where to go next.' And you ask for that bit of help and it's amazing how it comes. It might be in that moment, it might come later in the day, but inspiration does come."

John Parkin says of his own creativity, "I need to feel the tension of chaos. I need to feel the tension of something not being solved and not being worked out, and what I crave most is relief from that tension, and the moment of highest creativity – and this is liminal really – is the squeezing out of an idea, which is a relief from the chaos of not knowing. Creatively, the tension holds in it a desire for relief, of a door opening. I'm okay to be in that corridor space for a while, but then it's the relieving of the tension that is the creative moment for me."

Weave Wonder in a Story

All creatives – whether writers, artists, musicians, actors or sculptors – draw on their creativity to help us to make sense of the world. That is why we have such a strong emotional, and sometimes visceral, response to certain art forms that resonate with us. That's also why historically our forebears used the liminality of storytelling as a way to convey allegoric liminal life lessons; a story is a place where we are able to lose ourselves in the liminal space of not knowing how it will end, whether it's a book, film or other medium, and at the same time, the storyline can be a parable that helps to direct us and make sense of our lives.

Professional storyteller and author of *Be Your Own Fairytale: Working with story-telling for positive life change*, Alison Davies says, "The narrative allows us to feel that sense of wonder at not knowing what will come next, but we are able to do this in the safe space of the story. In real life, that feeling of uncertainty can be challenging and stressful, but in the framework of a story, it's exciting. We instantly put ourselves in that liminal space, which can be a thrilling experience. When we hear or read a story, we take the experiences and scenarios present to us and 'make it real' – this is a natural part of the process of connecting with the story.

"As we follow the narrative, in 'making the story real' for ourselves, we are able to experience the familiar and the unfamiliar just like the characters; the difference is that we are able to do this with some degree of detachment. Our logical mind knows the story isn't real, but we connect with the emotions, so it feels real. In effect, reading a story allows us to 'practise' and 'play out' different roles and scenarios so that we feel more comfortable when we do it for real in the world as is."

The classic vehicle for the storyline in any narrative is the premise of the Monomyth, or 'The Hero's Journey'. The term was coined by the American writer Joseph Campbell, who noticed that heroes in mythology typically go through the same three basic stages (and 17 detailed steps) in their journey to hero-dom. Namely they go on an adventure, face a crisis and win, then return victorious. He wrote about this in 1949 in his comparative mythology book *The Hero with a Thousand Faces*, which was later adapted into the TV show *The Power of Myth*. Despite its origins in ancient myths, it is still commonly used in modern-day adventure storytelling.

The stages of the Journey are: Act One starts at home or in a safe environment and at the end the protagonist decides to leave on a journey. In the second part, Act Two, s/he goes on a journey, often with an ally, where they meet an antagonist and there are challenges that must be overcome. Help comes from the ally but toward the end of Act Two, the obstacles appear insurmountable and our hero is in dire straits. In screenplay writing, this point in the story is known as the 'all is lost' moment. When it looks like the hero cannot win, the intractable difficulties are overcome, and in Act Three the protagonist and their ally return home, either literally or metaphorically, having learned something massive about themselves. You could view Act Two in any story as liminal space. It's where the protagonist starts to explore the wider world and/or themselves in greater depth and the outcome of the storyline is still uncertain.

John Parkin agrees, "Act Two, i.e., liminal space, is necessary for a journey of a life, but it's not always pleasant to be in. Yet, you can never get to Act Three without going through Act Two; you cannot get to the other side without the journey." Effectively, without the transformational possibilities of liminal space, our lives remain rooted in Act One – you stay at home.

Rites of Passage

Psychotherapist Michael Boyle is well aware of the transformational power of stories and he has been using storytelling in his rites of passage work with men, both young and old, for more than 20 years. He is a co-founder of the global The Mankind Project, which offers courses designed to help men to mentor each other to step out of their 'ordinary' life into an 'extra-ordinary' space, from where they are able to see themselves and their life with greater clarity. From that experience, Band of Brothers was born – a programme using rites of passage techniques to help younger men to negotiate the transition to better life choices for themselves, drawing on the wisdom, support and community of male elders who have been through The Mankind Project. Boyle says, "The Mankind Project and Band of Brothers experience rides on a story. I started off by telling the stories, and then we realized it is actually better to make a script out of them and to enact them with the men. It's an exacerbated liminal space because we go into this make-believe place. For us, liminal space is enhanced by the vehicle of the story. I'm guessing that was the way it always was when we were sitting around fires thousands of years ago. People were transported in their imagination and then that allowed new possibilities to open up.

"It's an eye-opener for the young men on the course that we actually involve them in stories. They always say, 'If you'd told me what was going to happen, I'd never have come. But I'm glad I did.' We set up very dramatic, powerful scenes, which you make your way through during the weekend. Then you spend the next few weeks in groups trying to work out what was going on for you. This integration part is really important. The elders have all been through the same thing, so there's nothing that goes on that they haven't been through, and when they're mentoring, there's a bond of the shared experience and a shared imagination that is very hard to get in the real world. Every experience has a physical, emotional, cognitive and imaginative/spiritual aspect to it that must be acknowledged. As a facilitator, you make sure all those bases are covered."

The Mankind Project and Band of Brothers were set up specifically to help men with some of life's more difficult transitions. For older men, this often happens as their children grow up and leave home, or they realize they've been doing an unrewarding job for years. It's classic midlife crisis stuff – the threat of death, divorce, disease – a wake-up call. As Boyle says, "They've lost that essential connection and feeling of contributing. They have insecurities around all sorts of things that the rite of passage relieves them of." For younger men, they may be exposed to pressure from gangs, or alcohol or drug misuse, law breaking or the feeling of not fitting in. Whatever it is, in both projects, the programme is designed to initiate them in a safe environment so they can cross the threshold from their old lives to a place of better self-understanding and growth.

"There are certain elements to a rite of passage that you have to include," explains Boyle. "There is the threshold – that movement from the ego, status, structured world into something unknown must be set up. Suddenly, life is not so familiar, there's disorientation – that's essential. That feeling of, 'I don't know where I am. I don't even know who I am. Nobody cares who I am. I definitely can't pull any status numbers or try to lord it over anybody else right here. That's not going to work.' And that's because there's an equality that happens in that space.

"Once there's this element of stepping over the threshold into the unknown, at that point, we've got the time in between what has passed and what's about to come. We are entering into a space of transition. There has to be a submission in the transition process – it's like a swan dive – giving yourself permission to let go. The men bring an emotional pain that has been taken on over years and they find out what it's about so that they can put it into some sort of context and get over it. The 'me too' thing is a really powerful positive part of it because when these young men (and it would be the same for young women too, I don't see any difference) come into these spaces, thinking that they're totally alone in their suffering and their pain, suddenly it's like, 'Whoa, me too,' and it's such a relief.

"We're here to let something die so that something can be born. That's really the essence of the transformational process. It's all reflection. We're in this place where we can reflect and pause." It is through putting themselves into this liminal state that those on the Mankind and Band of Brothers courses are able to afford themselves the essential suspended moment where self-discovery can dawn.

The Power of Ritual and the Experiential

Throughout history, initiations and rites of passage were an essential milestone in a young person's life, marking the transition from callow youth to responsible adult, or in the case of young men, perhaps to warrior. These rituals marked an individual's transition from one social or religious status to another. So, the stages of life were celebrated – such as the birth of a child, a youth's coming of age or the funeral of a respected member of the family or community, as well as movement through the ranks of the existing priesthoods.

Across the ancient world, boys were forced to prove their "manliness" with tough, often bloody, rituals. Some societies demanded bloodshed to mark this major milestone in life, others demanded shows of obedience or bravery. For centuries, a coming-of-age ritual for the young men of the island of Vanuatu was an early form of bungee jumping – using two tree vines attached to the ankle and jumping off a 30-foot wooden platform – to test the courage of the individual and to mark his passage into adulthood. The ancient Aboriginal peoples in Australia had a number of painful ways for boys to prove their manhood, culminating in a 'knocking out' ceremony, which involved the initiate's tooth being knocked out with a rock and handed to his mother. And, for the ancient Mongols, a boy would have to learn how to hunt with eagles before he joined the men of his tribe. Meanwhile, some early societies simply required a symbolic change in hairstyle or clothing. In ancient Rome, for example, progressing to a plain white toga for a young boy at the age of around 12–13 years old was a symbolic move into manhood, and in the Confucian *Guan Li* ceremony in ancient China, a young man's hair was ceremonially cut and a change of clothes took place.

What these ceremonies all have in common is that there is an element of uncertainty built in. The liminal phase in the middle of the ritual, helps underline the importance of the transition, and offers the initiate a chance to contemplate and digest the meaning of this change in status. Although historically, many rites of passage involved hard physical challenges, according to the school of social science known as structural functionalism, they also served to relieve the stress that individuals feel when they enter the liminal space of great changes or rearrangements that occur in their lives, and they provide instruction in and approval of the new roles that may arise through such occasions.

I have long been a huge fan of respected healer, teacher and author of *Quest: A Guide For Creating Your Own Vision Quest* Denise Linn, ever since I attended one of her courses many years ago. She is of Native American heritage and used to run vision quests. A vision quest usually involves going into nature alone, often with the support of a group/community to which you return, and seeking to tap into the unseen wisdom all around and inside you. In that liminal state, you can make space for your own hero's journey to unfold. She explains that the process of leaving the comfort of your environment behind and venturing beyond what is safe and secure for you, namely into the liminal, is a key element. Traditionally, a vision quest lasts around three to four days, usually without food, and it would be considered as a rite of passage to mark big life changes and to shift you into a place of better self-knowledge.

She says, "In native tradition, it is usually held at a time where a young woman or young man goes into puberty, because that is the time when they are starting to get clarity about what their life will be as an adult. But for us, in Western culture, it can be at any time. It's like answering the call. You can be 65 years old and you get the call. What is the call? Well, it's this yearning. You know something needs to change. It can come literally at any time. It's not about the physicalness of your life. It's more in the realm of your soul. The important thing is to listen. So often people say, 'Well, I don't have time for it,' or 'I can't do it now. Maybe next year.' But, if you can just skid to a halt and say, 'Okay, I heard you, and I'm ready,' that decision, even before you go on a quest, that's the point of power, because you're listening."

Historically, the end of a rite of passage was marked by some ritual practice or challenge that was witnessed by the whole community. Obviously, that is not something that can happen in modern society, so I ask Michael Boyle if there is a modern substitute for the traditional community recognition and approbation. He feels it is as important as ever that the initiates on the courses are acknowledged, recognized and witnessed by the group. He says, "There is A Band of Brothers community and there's also a Mankind Project community. During the weekend, we work with the shadow stuff, obviously, and all the bits of them that undermine their best interest, but eventually, they are witnessed in their 'gold', in their quality [at their best] and that is key, for the youngsters in particular. That public recognition thing is a really vital part of it."

Given that it is hard to simulate the community recognition element of a rite of passage in the modern world, and that it takes some courage to set out on a quest where you don't know how you might fare or what awaits you on the other side – as Denise Linn states, "a quest of any kind is a heroic journey" – I wondered why you'd put yourself through that. In the past, a vision quest was a rite of passage and a doorway to the spiritual realm, but what might be the motivation for a modern-day quest? Linn says, "It's not so much a goal as just wanting to stop. Stopping the treadmill of life, just stopping that constant hum. It's like when you're in a room for a long time with the air conditioning unit running – you don't actually hear the air conditioner until it stops. And when it stops, there's this inhalation, and this 'Ah!' moment. When people are drawn to quest, I don't know that they're thinking, 'Oh, I want to have visions.' I think it's more a deep yearning for that place of stillness; a deep yearning for the hum to stop. In that hum stopping, in that solitude, in that silence, then you can hear your own voice, the voice of your soul, as you can't usually hear it. I often think of driving at night-time across the desert on a lonely stretch of road, and you can only get static on the radio. You get used to it being just static, but if you just tune it a little bit, one way or the other, you can get this crystal-clear channel. For me, a quest is being able to tune that dial just a tiny bit so you can hear that beautiful clarity of spirit, which is really hard to hear when you're in the 'doingness' of life.

"When you're in the midst of your everyday life, it's really difficult to get into that place of stillness because the physical patterns of thinking and doing run so deep. In native cultures, they knew and understood this. They understood that a young man or young woman literally had to leave the tribe, had to be out in a different environment, in order to hear, in order to see, in order to feel, in order to know the truth of their soul."

Experiential Learning

I was curious as to how rites of passage therapies differ from talking therapies, for example, and Michael Boyle explained that the experiential and ritualistic elements of the experience play a major role, in addition to the mentoring and integration aspects. He points out to me, "The powerful thing about the liminal space is that it's an experience, which is special. Most of the schooling we have now is all about taking in information and regurgitating it back. You're informed, but you don't learn much. We learn best through experiences. When it's experiential, the messages stick with you and then you can self-reflect. In many ways, the rite of passage is offering people, especially the young men, in a safe environment, an opportunity for self-reflection, for revelations about themselves, but also, alongside that, the comfort of knowing that they're not alone, that they're not the only person who feels this way or thinks that way."

In his classic 1909 book, *The Rites of Passage*, the French ethnographer Arnold van Gennep who first coined the phrase, described rites of passage as having three phases: separation, liminality and incorporation, and he puts a great deal of emphasis on the importance of the rituals and ceremonies that mark someone's new status before integration into the 'post-liminal' new world.

Eliana Harvey has been running the Shamanka retreats in the Dorset countryside for over 20 years to reconnect women with their ancient potency and to coach them in personal and environmental healing. It is the only internationally known school dedicated uniquely to women's shamanism (traditionally a shaman, who could be male or female, used trance to achieve various powers including healing the sick, communicating with the otherworld and escorting the souls of the dead). It has been her personal quest to recover and reweave the ancient shamanic knowledge and the hidden teachings of the women's mysteries.

Whenever I have met Eliana, I have always been impressed by the powerful presence she emits and the great wisdom that she is so willing to share. She is a great believer in the power of ritual. On her courses, women make full use of ceremonies involving fire, dance and drumming. She says, "Ritual and ceremony, as well as the sacrificial stuff, which is very important, because it involves body movement, very often takes in every part of you, so it can be more potent than just talking therapies, or intellectual conceptions. Ritual reaches every part of you and, because it involves the whole being, it goes deeply into the subconscious. Using symbols, it bypasses the normal, literal function of the mind and emotions. The dominant part of the brain is logical, yet the role that ritual plays is not logical. It has a different energy. Ritual goes to that deeper part of ourselves, to that deep intuitive part that women automatically have. It's our greatest gift."

Being Present

Considering the difficulties most people have in embracing the unknown, I am struck by the contradictory nature of our lives when considered in the light of Robert Holden's belief that we are all afflicted by 'destination addiction', that too many of us spend our lives suspended in limbo looking to a brighter, happier future. I talked with him about why some people tend toward nostalgia, thinking that life was better in the past – the Paradise Lost approach – while others tend to look forward, always thinking there's this utopia that they haven't yet reached – Ithaca. Holden suggests, "We are not taught to have much trust or faith in the present moment. Our work is always about getting to a better now, rather than being in this now. We promise ourselves that when we do find our amazing now, we'll really slow down, we'll really be more present, we'll be more engaged, more mindful. And we mean that in good faith. But the point is that no *now* will be enough if you're not present. If you're not there, any now you find yourself in is always going to feel like something is missing in your life.

"What I learned in my own life – and this took quite a while – was that I was always haunted by the feeling that something was missing in my life, and that's what fuelled my own destination addiction, because I was more into getting there than being here. Eventually, it dawned on me little by little, that maybe what was missing from my life was me. So, if you think something's missing in your life, maybe it's *you*, more of your connection to your heart, more of the soulful you, more of the real you rather than the frantic you, the hectic you, the you that says you'll relax when you get there. If you give *now* more of a chance, the now that you're in will become more interesting. If you're more present to the now you're in, if you inhabit this now, it's going to feel less empty, it's going to feel like it's got a gift for you, a lesson for you, a sign for you."

Paradoxically, it seems that constantly putting life on hold awaiting the perfect timing to live our best lives is unwittingly keeping us in a different kind of liminal suspension. How many times do you tell yourself that once you reach this goal, get that promotion, gain this qualification or live in that place that things will be better and you can really start to live life fully? This belief that life over the hill will be fuller and more rewarding is what is preventing us from making the very most of what we are experiencing at present. Holden told me, "There is a lot of searching – searching for happiness, looking for love, hoping to find our purpose, the quest for greater wisdom. We're always searching – which is vital to get us going – but at a certain point too much searching probably suggests that we're experiencing some sort of blindness. I think what happens when we're in liminal space is that we exchange searching for *being*, and that's part of the work. In the liminal space, we have to let ourselves be lost so we can be guided. When we're in the darkness, we've got to give up hope because when you're in the liminal space, you're often hoping for the wrong things. Basically, what you're hoping is that your original plan or life will get reinstated. Understandably, we're lost and we're going, 'I need my original life back and, if I hope enough, it'll happen.' But actually, you've almost got to give up all hopes for your original plan working.

"One thing I find is that your positivity isn't helpful in the liminal space very often. I always say that emotional honesty trumps positivity really. If you try to be too positive, you end up getting lost in the liminal space for longer. You almost have to ditch your positivity and be emotionally honest. If you do that about where you are, you get more clarity. If you pretend to be all right where you are, that blocks your receptors. You have to learn to be able to say, 'Look, I am lost, and I'm scared, but I'm open. I've given up all hope, and I have faith.'

It's that sort of in between, where you're cultivating a quality that is sometimes called equanimity. By being honest, a new positivity emerges. It's a light that you're not trying to generate, it's more a light that comes to you. It comes back to basic trust that I am in the right place. It's appropriate that I don't know where I am right now. I'm probably between chapters. I might even be between stories. I do think people are getting two or three lifetimes for the price of one these days."

Now he's lost me. Does he mean we are more likely to have portfolio careers now? Is that what he's getting at? I ask for greater clarification and he expands, "I get a feeling that we seem to shake up our lives or we have our lives shaken up more often, you know, like two or three times in a lifetime. The rate we get through marriages and divorces, but also definitely in our careers. Liminal space, being in that in between, is something we're having to learn to address more and more."

Liminal Life Lessons

Although our default setting as humans is security and homeostasis, it seems clear that retaining that status quo can limit our potential for self-discovery, creativity and determining what truly makes us happy. By putting ourselves into liminal space, not necessarily to the extremes that some of our interviewees have gone to but certainly taking time out for reflection and review, perhaps with the aid of talking therapy, a course or a rite of passage/quest, then we open ourselves to greater possibilities and potential.

Certainly, if transition is thrust upon us, as it almost certainly will be at various points in our lives, although it may be challenging, these liminal periods can be immense growth opportunities. If, at these times, we accept that this is where we find ourselves and take time to take stock – how does this uncertainty feel in our body, emotions and mind? It is necessary to remind ourselves that we are okay in this moment, rather than slipping into catastrophic thinking about what might happen, and then it can be a positive opening to other options.

Here is some guidance and advice that our experts have gleaned through personal experience or in their professional lives as coaches, which I hope you find inspirational. I also have 'take-aways' from the chapter – personal reflections and suggestions that I have gathered from my writing of this chapter or practices that I use in my everyday life that you might also find helpful.

Expert Inspiration #One

Abigail Bergstrom, who consciously chose to let go of everything that was familiar in her life, says, "I stopped reading and listening to podcasts. I watched very little cinema. I just completely closed off from all external sources. For me, it was about just sitting with myself. It's almost like you have to take a step back and remove yourself from your life in order to get the bird's eye view and see what's going on. Being so anchorless, the only solution is to turn in and reconnect with yourself and I think that makes for creativity. When I was in that liminal place in my life, I was painting and drawing, and I felt like I really was connecting with my child self, who was like, 'Please, more play, more fun, more lightness.'"

Expert Inspiration #Two

John Parkin shared from his F**k It courses, "When we invite people to say F**k It to things, we are asking them to trust themselves and to move into the territory that's not the predicted. You have to step into the unknown.

"First of all, you open to new stuff and new ideas. Secondly, you relax because the intuition that we tune into from relaxation is different to the intuition from tension, which is mainly fear-based. So, you have to relax. Then, you tune in to what's coming up. It's a kind of relistening or moving the weight or the centre of gravity of listening from the outside world to the inside world. Ask yourself, 'What's really going on here? What would I like to be doing? How would I like to spend my time? Even this afternoon and this evening, not just in my life.' Then you trust that the messages you're getting are really powerful and you follow those powerful messages."

Expert Inspiration #Three

Talking about the liminal space of transition, Michael Boyle says, "Life's transitions come constantly, don't they? I encourage people to ask themselves, 'What is the way of being that you're leaving behind? And what is the way of being you're moving into?' And you can use archetypes to experience that and rehearse it, so that you can anchor it.

"Sometimes, we need someone holding the context, what I might call a ritual elder, to take us into another space, beyond what we thought we were capable of. You can't always do that on your own. So that's why people go off on retreats and meditate, or go into therapy. It's all liminal space and I don't think there's any substitute for entering into a space of transition, liminal space, where the agenda is the transformational process."

Expert Inspiration #Four

Denise Linn also feels that having someone experienced with you on a quest can be helpful, although not essential. She says, "There is value in having someone present as a sacred observer, a sacred witness if you will, someone who understands the things that can come up. In the quests that I lead, people make their own sacred circle and they would designate it, they would honour it and they would cherish it. That was to create a sense of safety, because it's not uncommon when you're on these quests to get really scared. It can be terrifying to be confronted with the vast wholeness of yourself, or when you're confronted with your fear it's an opportunity to step beyond it. So, having someone there, even if they're not in your circle, knowing that there's someone there who understands that it is a courageous journey that you're on can make it easier.

Nonetheless, you can get the same results yourself, which is one of the reasons why I wrote *Quest*, so that people begin to understand all the forces at play if they do decide to do it themselves."

Expert Inspiration #Five

In naming 'destination addiction', namely the way that he was always getting to a destination only to create the next, Robert Holden realized that it was fundamentally an unkind experience. To help others to avoid this, he recommends, "Cultivate a better relationship to now. Ask yourself the questions, 'How could I enjoy now more? What good things could come about in my life if I were more present? What good things might happen if I was more focussed on now, rather than the future?' Why not write a question at the top of a blank page or in a notebook and listen to your inner voice? I have great faith in questions and I think we carry the answers within us. We know our truth voice. The bottom line is that the future is just made up of more 'now' anyway – so you don't change the future in the future, you change the future in the present."

My Chapter Take-aways

- Despite our dislike and mistrust of change, there are bound to be periods of unplanned transition in our lives, so we need to get comfortable with them. Why not try putting yourself into situations that are slightly outside your comfort zone, or where the outcome is unknown to you. Of course, putting yourself into liminal space does not have to be as extreme as giving up your job or selling your home. Take a solitary hike or city break in a new destination – spending time alone is revealing. Start a new challenging hobby or join a club. Volunteer. In this way, you can build up your tolerance to new experiences and thus handle any unexpected change that may be thrust on you, in a much calmer manner. There are so many different ways to experiment and explore the liminal in our lives; I highly recommend it. It's in these moments, in the gap in between, that the real personal growth and self-discovery takes place.

- It can help to attend a workshop, take a course or to see a talking therapist as a catalyst for change. Through my career as a journalist, I have been lucky enough to attend many self-development courses ranging from physical outdoor challenge-style courses through to the purely theoretical mindfulness workshops. All take you away from your normal environment and, while you are suspended in a liminal middle space, the facilitators skilfully lead you toward an opportunity for self-discovery, self-truth and new realizations.

- We can spend much of our lives in limbo by nostalgically dwelling in the past or thinking life will be better/easier in the future, rather than living our best life in the present. When you catch yourself in this habit, try to bring yourself back to the present and appreciate what you have now. I do a daily gratitude practice. It's nothing fancy and you can do it any time of day. Often, just before I fall asleep at night, I silently list a few of the things that have happened or I've noticed during the day for which I am thankful, or that simply brightened my day. Being appreciative helps you to make the most of the life you're living right now.

- On a yoga and meditation retreat in Thailand run by inspirational teacher Brett Moran, author of *Wake the F**k Up*, I learned a fantastic practice that helps to combat catastrophic thinking – one of the biggest obstacles to taking a chance and putting yourself into new and unknown liminal situations. When you catch yourself spiralling down into negative 'What if' thinking – What if I can't do it? What if they don't like me? What if I get it wrong? – play the 'What if Up' game. Ask yourself – What if it goes really well, where might that lead me? What if I meet some new people who introduce me to a broader network? What if I get it right and my new business flies? This game is a great way to motivate yourself to do the things that scare you and to take a leap into the liminal unknown.

2

HOVERING BETWEEN LIFE AND DEATH

For me, the most obvious, and certainly the most extreme, example of being on the threshold, of entering into liminality, is the process of passing from this life into whatever lies on the other side. When we hover on the brink between living and dying, we are in a liminal space.

Most of us are uncomfortable around death, and many of us have a strange suspicion that if we talk about death, we might invite it into our lives sooner than it needs to be, which is a great shame because the more we can talk about it and make it a part of life, the more we can be at ease with it, the less fearful we will become and the more likely we are to have the kind of death that we would want for ourselves and/or our loved ones.

Until the mid-20th century, most people still died at home with neighbours and relatives in the house, so we knew what death looked, sounded and smelled like, which in a way prepared us all eventually for our own passing, because it was familiar and normal. Now, most people die in hospital, or perhaps a hospice, and they're looked after by other people with a lot of machinery around them, and we don't know what to do or say anymore. Most importantly, we've lost the ability to recognize the stages of death that our loved ones pass through. Of course, cultures vary in how death is conceptualized and marked. In Western cultures, death is said to occur only when there is a total cessation of life. Some cultural traditions view death as a transition to other forms of existence, such as in the Christian faith where the person sheds their bodily form and continues on in spirit; others propose a continuous interaction between the dead and the living, such as among some Native American tribes and certain segments of Buddhism. Some cultures conceive a circular pattern of multiple deaths and rebirths as in Hinduism; and yet atheists view death as the final end, with nothing occurring after it. Despite this broad spectrum of beliefs, the actual process of dying is still something that mystifies us.

If anyone can shed light on the passage from life into death, it would be Felicity Warner, a 'soul midwife' who has lovingly witnessed countless passings in a career spanning more than 25 years. She has made it her life's mission to study the dying process, not only so she can help others to die with dignity and love, and in the best way possible for them, but also to help the anguished families who so often find themselves in a state of confusion and helplessness as their loved ones are dying, frequently in a hospital bed and removed from them.

Her quest started when, at the age of 13, she was kept apart from the grandmother who had raised her as the old lady was dying alone in hospital from lung cancer.

The whole harrowing episode left an indelible mark on Warner, who, although staying with a neighbour, felt an ecstatic moment of peaceful release at the exact time her grandmother died in hospital; a fact that she only found out the next morning. At the time, she didn't understand it, but with the benefit of years of being with people as they die, she now explains it by saying, "When we are very closely connected with another, we can almost share that moment of relief, if you like. In some ways, it's a gift the dying can give to the living. I really was experiencing how it was for her to escape that cancer-ridden body that was no longer supporting her in any way at all."

In her mid-thirties, Warner was working as a journalist with a group of women of a similar age to herself who were all dying from breast cancer, and who wanted their experiences to be recorded. "It was their stories that really woke me up and made me realize how badly we do death and how awkward, inadequate and fearful we feel with dying people. I then started volunteering in hospices, and I realized that if we bring together things such as complementary medicine and spirituality alongside their clinical care, in a very loose and gentle way, we offer people so much more."

Having worked exclusively since then with the dying, I asked her whether she had noticed any signs of a transition phase as people pass from life to death, and what she thought this liminal state might be like for them. She says, "I'm fascinated by the three days leading up to death and the three days after death, because they're so rich in the process that people go through. The things I've seen to support that have given me such insights about that transitionary state. Putting it in a nutshell, as people become more poorly and their bodies are deteriorating, they start to blossom on a spiritual level – there's a sort of dynamic shift. For many, the body is getting weak but, inside, there's something like a quickening really and, being trained, I can see this happening.

"When people are on the cusp of leaving this world, it's as if their field extends and they become much more sensitive to things, almost as if they are inhabiting two worlds at the same time. So, they often see people that we don't see, and they'll often have a conversation with someone who you can't see in the room, but the conversation is full of clarity and utterly extraordinary. They may see lights and colours. This is well-documented, and I just see it as them extending their vibrational range really. You get this real kind of in-between threshold energy and threshold experience. It can be a wonderful stage for people; not everybody, but most people, in my experience. Some who experience these states are incredibly calmed by them and reassured. It's the most wonderful thing to watch."

From my own understanding of sitting with my dear old dad at the end, I saw him fighting death all the way, so I can't help thinking that it's not like this for everyone. Warner acknowledges that there are occasions where people have no apparent trips into this liminal space, or even that they may have more disturbing visions and reactions to being in these in-between places. Often in those situations, although by no means always, the person who is dying has unfinished business in their life with no chance or time to resolve that, she tells me.

Obviously it's not news that we shouldn't wait until someone is on their death bed before telling them the things that we want them to hear. We should strive to make our peace with friends and family at every stage of our lives, to ensure we have no outstanding issues – not just getting our affairs in order in terms of financial administration, but also our relationships. Warner agrees, and suggests that we be more mindful of the Native American saying: "Today is a good day to die, for everything is in place."

I asked her what other observations she had taken from a lifetime of caring for the dying? She says, "I suppose, because I hear more stories about death than most people, I'm conscious of the fact that life is fragile, so I never take it for granted. Every day is a precious and beautiful day, and even if it's not looking like a great day, I will try and unpick the wonderful bits about it and practise gratitude. I have seen enough people before and slightly after death to believe that actually, it isn't the end. There is so much more that comes afterwards, but it is the great mystery. None of us absolutely know for sure, so we have to surrender to that mystery.

"It's not as though enlightenment has come to me as of yet, but I live in hope. There's a lot to be said about treating people as you wish to be treated yourself – just trying to be kind and help others. At the end of the day it probably boils down to having a compassionate heart and being comfortable in your own skin."

A Trial Run: Near Death Experiences

Since Felicity Warner told me that the dying spend a lot of time going in and out of their bodies, "It's almost as if they're practising being there, but not being there – as if they're not fully present and grounded in their bodies", as she puts it – it got me thinking about the sorts of experiences that people report when they talk about having an Out of Body Experience (OBE), or a Near Death Experience (NDE) as the liminal space between life and death, given that NDE and OBE experiencers live to tell the tale.

NDE and OBE experiences most commonly occur while the person is in a life and death situation, often in hospital undergoing emergency surgery or in intensive care. This led me to meet with Penny Sartori who worked as a hospital nurse for 21 years, 17 of those in intensive care units. Having sat with a man who experienced a lonely and particularly difficult passing, Sartori began to question the process of death itself and, with the permission of the hospital authorities, she began to investigate the transition into death more fully. In 2005, she was awarded a PhD for her extensive research into NDEs and she has also published three books on the subject, the latest of which is *The Transformative Powers of Near-Death Experiences: How the Messages of NDEs Positively Impact the World.*

Sartori conducted her PhD study over five years, interviewing patients who had survived their admission to the intensive care unit. Once recovering, she would ask them if they had any memories of the time that they were unconscious. Most initially were suspicious of her motives and somewhat noncommittal, but when she explained that she had a deep interest in what people experience, they started to open up. She says, "For many, they didn't understand their experience. They were overwhelmed by it, because they had no point of reference for it. It was unlike any other human experience they'd ever had before. So, by talking and asking questions, it was really helpful to process what had happened to them.

"One of the most common themes that they reported was meeting deceased relatives or friends, who told them that it wasn't their time, that they had to go back. What I found slightly different to the reports I'd read about in the general NDE literature was that some of these relatives or friends were quite angry, saying, 'You shouldn't be here, go back,' as if scolding them, and I'd not come across that before. Some of them went to beautiful gardens or another realm, and many had overwhelming feelings of peace, joy and calm. A few had a life review and some had Out of Body Experiences where they found themselves looking down on their own bodies."

Sartori found that most people change quite profoundly after an NDE, especially with regards to their values. Many take on a more spiritual approach to life, to the extent that they can no longer feel aligned with their old job and many change careers, often opting for the caring professions or carrying out voluntary work. Sadly, this sudden and drastic change in outlook and attitude can be upsetting or confusing for loved ones, and NDE experiencers often report that this can result in relationship issues.

Since an NDE is such an amazing life-altering experience, I am surprised to learn that many people who experience one are not sure about what has happened to them.

"Most didn't realize that they'd had an NDE because they didn't understand it," she says. "The majority of people never volunteer the information. I only came across the people in my study because I was doing my research and I'd asked them. Out of the 15 cases that I had in my first research group, only two people had volunteered that information. If I hadn't asked if they had any recall of the time they were unconscious, 13 people would never have discussed it with me or anyone else."

Current estimates for NDEs among all people who are successfully resuscitated hover between 11 and 20 per cent, according to Sartori, but given her findings, it would seem to imply that NDEs and OBEs are more prevalent than these statistics suggest.

One of the main reasons people don't discuss their NDEs and OBEs is clearly because they don't know what they are, but also, we might assume that many worry about telling people about such experiences and attracting derision. They know that something amazing has happened but they can't make any sense of it – and many ascribe the experience to the drugs they've been given or to hallucinations, Sartori tells me.

Pinch Me, I'm Dreaming

In point of fact, that didn't sound like such an unreasonable explanation to me, and many medics and scientists dismiss patient accounts of these phenomena as just that – a hallucination. So, I asked how we could be sure that the liminal space entered in an NDE is not just a figment of a dream or hallucination, or some type of drug-induced experience? Sartori says, "I did look at hallucinations as well in my research and I documented cases of those. I analysed them and got very different findings. When I followed up with the patients who had been hallucinating, they could rationalize that it was an hallucination – they knew. In the cases of the hallucinations, they might involve things that were going on in the background as they were waking up from sedation. So, you could attribute them to the things that were actually being done to the patients, and the conversations they could hear and the noises in the room.

"By contrast, those who had an NDE were adamant that it was real, in fact realer than real, asserting that unless you've had the experience yourself, you can't possibly understand it. Not only were the two experiences very different, but one patient in my study, while he was deeply unconscious and having an NDE, communicated with a deceased member of his family, who gave him information that only one living member of the family could know. When he later told the relative, she was astounded because that information is something that she had gone to great lengths to hide from him and to keep secret."

Certainly, garnering unknowable and indisputable facts from a relative that you met in an NDE that are later verified by a living person strikes me as a difficult thing to explain away by the hallucination theory. But is there any more compelling evidence?

I turned to Dr Eben Alexander, a renowned neurological surgeon who himself had an NDE during a week-long coma following a devastating attack on his brain from bacterial meningitis, which is almost always a death sentence. In his book *Living in a Mindful Universe: A Neurosurgeon's Journey into the Heart of Consciousness* (the follow-up to his bestseller *Proof of Heaven: A neurosurgeon's journey into the afterlife* describing his NDE experience), he offers a powerful scientific version of an understanding of reality where consciousness is fundamental – a conclusion he reached as a result of his own experience and subsequent research. He explains, "Materialist scientists would say, 'Our theories don't allow for something like an NDE, so they're all made-up nonsense.' Well, tell that to the 13 million Americans who have had an NDE. You've got to reverse a tremendous amount of misguided thinking and faulty assumptions around the evidence. Those who claim to be sceptics are, for the most part, pseudosceptics. They have made up their mind. They believe the materialist worldview and they see no way that that worldview can explain how these kinds of events can happen. So, they ignore empirical data and they don't care about rational argument."

So, how would he debunk the hallucination explanation that is so often used by the materialist sceptics to counter NDE claims? Firstly, he says that the case report on his own NDE that was published in *The Journal of Nervous and Mental Disease* in September 2018 made it very clear that his neocortex was inactivated and his brain was in no shape to support any kind of dream or hallucination at all. He then falls back on empirical evidence to support this, saying, "It's become very clear, in NDE literature, that one of the things that's so shocking about NDE memories is they don't change. They're kind of burned in forever. Normally, every time you return to a memory, you alter it a little bit. That's not the case with NDE memories. They're very vivid, crisp, real. In fact, my memories of my NDE are as sharp today as if they happened yesterday. And there's another aspect to it; for the 36 hours after I was extubated after I woke up from coma, my brain was still just frazzled with the whole experience. I had these kind of paranoid, delusional psychotic nightmares known as an ICU psychosis. I was in and out of awareness in the ICU, and just crazy in between times.

"As much as I initially bundled all the memories together – the ultra-real spiritual memories from the NDE together with the post-coma craziness – the post-trauma craziness memories disappeared, even though I wrote them down and tried to remember them to tell that story. They're nothing more than a covered over memory, as opposed to the rich, ultra-real spiritual memories from deep in the NDE.

"There are several papers from Dr Bruce Grayson, one of the world's leading medical experts on NDEs, and other sources showing that the consistency and resilience of NDE memories are much more like real lived events than any kind of imaginary or dream event or hallucination. So, there's something very special and powerful about them."

Leaping into the Unknown – Voluntary OBEs

While most NDEs happen spontaneously and under extreme circumstances, that is not always the case with Out of Body Experiences (OBEs). There are widely known ethnographical reports of shamans purposely leaving their body during trance or sleep to meet with the ancestors or spirits, and some people claim to be able to voluntarily and repeatedly induce OBEs for themselves.

Before pursuing that line of enquiry, I wanted to know what the definition for an Out of Body experience actually was. In this instance, I turned to medical anthropologist Samantha Lee Treasure, who is researching OBEs as part of her PhD thesis and is herself an OBE experiencer since childhood. She explains that, "OBEs are experiences in which you have a sensation or perception of being outside of your physical body. And you could say the same about dreams in a way, but there are a number of differences. For example, classic dreams occur in REM sleep, and OBEs are either during sleep, but not necessarily the REM stage, or while awake, but normally when doing repetitive activities, or when stressed physically, emotionally or mentally."

I wondered how this differed from a lucid dream, for example. It transpires that Treasure has asked this very question of the participants in her study. She says, "I asked them how they distinguish between OBEs and lucid dreams, as they both involve wake-like cognition. The main answer given to me by all of the participants was the transition state that often precedes the OBE, and it's normally quite jarring and frightening, especially the first time it happens. It can involve really intense physical sensations, such as vibrating or shaking and being pulled out of body as well. There are also really intense sounds that sometimes accompany the transition, like mechanical sounds, bangs or buzzing, and sometimes there are voices. If this process doesn't frighten them too much and is allowed to continue, this would initiate an Out of Body Experience proper where they would feel themselves to be floating or pulled out, and these transition sensations would fade away.

"The other feature of the OBE that they commented on was how realistic it feels compared to dreams. It generally occurs in a realistic facsimile of an environment, and it's very stable, logical and progresses along linear time rather than jumping from scene to scene, or being fantastical like in dreams. They can have a very clear recall of OBEs as well, and they feel very immersive."

She also told me that some OBE experiencers find themselves returning to the same locations time and time again, "Some people say that when they have an OBE, they can think of a place and they can go there. But for me, most of the time, I am pulled somewhere; and 80–90% of the time, I get pulled to this location that seems very realistic and it always seems the same. This sounds crazy, but it seems like Tokyo in the future. And most of the time, I'm in another body or in another person."

Given the fact that the OBEs she described sounded pretty scary to me – one study by Susan Blackmore found about 25% of the general population have a negative OBE – I was curious to know why OBE experiencers were so keen to voluntarily repeat the experience. What did they discover in this unknown liminal world that was so compelling?

After some reflection, and it was clearly difficult for her to articulate, Treasure says, "It's a sense of exploration that humans have. We want to go to new territories on Earth and outside of Earth. These OBE spaces are like that too. It feels like you're going into a different environment and you're exploring a new plane. It's really hard to explain, but it feels like a different terrain, like an unexplored, unchartered territory. I think a lot of it is that desire for exploration."

That kind of makes sense to me. It's like the answer to the eternal question, why do you climb mountains? Because they're there. So, I can see why those who have had an OBE might want to explore this new liminal realm more fully. Yet, voluntary OBEs, given that no-one fully understands what liminal space you are entering, still sound rather risky to me.

I put this to Treasure and she agrees that certain precautions and prior research into teachers' credentials is required before experimenting with self-induced OBEs. She tells me about a shaman who was used to going into a trance and leaving his body. This particular shaman told one of Treasure's associates that he would never tell somebody to just walk into a jungle that they've never walked into before and to just embrace it; that would be irresponsible. He said that you should learn how to navigate it and that the astral realm is the same. In this regard, Treasure feels the same way and believes that if you are keen to experience an OBE for yourself, then you should research the course or instructors well before committing, as so many workshops have sprung up recently. To her, community is the most important recommendation she can make – joining a group or an online forum to talk about your OBE experience with other experiencers can be really useful.

While there are precautions you can take before voluntarily inducing an OBE experience, more people have a spontaneous OBE, and reports abound of hospital patients looking down on their own body from the corner of the room while the medics scurry around them, before they re-enter their body. However, these OBE reports are usually from the sleep or unconscious state. So, it was surprising to me that a spontaneous OBE can happen when you're awake.

It seems that OBEs can occur while awake as the result of a number of causes, including trauma, illness, drug use, extreme exercise or meditation practice, and that they occur in 10-20 per cent of the general healthy population, at least in Western or industrialized societies. What I found particularly fascinating is that, according to Treasure, "It happens to athletes or people rock climbing, for example. There are a few different researchers who have said that it could be that when you look at a room, if you took a picture of your view, it would be in 2D. But the brain maps a 3D structure in the head, like a model. So, we all have models of our environment. So, if you slip when you're rock climbing, perhaps because you're tired, and you might be seriously injured, or worse, suddenly you can have an out of body experience. People report that, most of the time, in that state, they have either no emotion or they have a kind of blissful feeling. In most of the accounts I've read like this, where it's a life-or-death situation, they generally feel suddenly very calm, and the one thing people say across the board is that their mind feels clearer than it ever has. They can see from outside the situation. So, they then have the time and the capacity to go, 'Oh, I need to reach up to that rock there.' And then, whoosh, they're back in their body knowing what to do."

What is this Space Between Life and Death?

It's not known whether the astral realm that is accessed during OBEs is the same space as that visited in NDEs or during the dying process – what or where is this liminal place that people visit? I'm familiar with the Tibetan Buddhist concept of *bardo*, the notion of a transitional process that usually refers to the gap between lives. Buddhists are masters of the art of caring for those who are dying and newly dead and they have practices that Felicity Warner and her soul midwives have adopted.

The Tibetan word 'Bardo' is translated as 'gap, interval, intermediate state, transitional process, or in between' and in Mahayana Buddhism usually refers to the gap between lives. According to the Tibetan teachings (Tibet is a Mahayana country), there are three death bardos: the painful bardo of dying, the luminous bardo of dharmata, and the karmic bardo of becoming.

When Buddhists in Mahayana countries are dying, someone whispers the name of the Buddha into their ear so that this is the last thing the person hears before they die. After death, relatives wash the body. They then place the body in a coffin surrounded by wreaths and candles. The funeral often takes place a few days after the death to allow the first bardo state to happen. This is the time when the dead person becomes conscious of being dead and the next form of rebirth is decided. Buddhists in Mahayana countries think that rebirth takes up to 49 days (7 weeks) after death. So, for those seven weeks, detailed guidance is read to the dead person from an appropriate text, such as *The Tibetan Book of the Dead,* to help them to pass through the intermediate bardo states.

I ask Felicity Warner about this bardo state in the dying process, as witnessed and supported by her and her soul midwives. She describes what happens immediately after someone passes, "Death may have been noted but there's a subtle acknowledgement that consciousness is still there. Very calmly, very kindly and with a lot of compassion, using heart energy, we say something such as, 'Don't worry, you're loved, you're supported, you're no longer of your body but you are in the light,' or 'you are spirit,' whatever is the right sort of thing to say for that person. Then we always light a candle and hold space while this subtle, I call it 'the unbinding', takes place. This goes back to our soul midwives' model of how we see consciousness after death. We see two energies unwinding away from each other, one is spirit and one is soul. Spirit is to do with who we've been in this lifetime. The soul energy unbinding in the other direction is the eternal aspect of who we are. It is infinite. We see these two energies pulling apart and that takes around three days to happen so we honour it, and we can do that even if a body has been taken down to the mortuary after death."

Penny Sartori believes that scientific advances help us to have a better understanding of the liminal transition between life and death, "Our science and our technology are becoming much more advanced and many more people are surviving a cardiac arrest or a close brush with death. So, there are more people having Near Death Experiences, and we're learning from these people. I think we're coming full circle because it's taking us back to the roots of the wisdom traditions.

"So, if someone has flatlined, their heart isn't beating and their brain is not receiving oxygen, to all intents and purposes, they should not be having any conscious experience at all. But people who have NDEs seem to be in a heightened state of consciousness. To me, it's more logical that consciousness is primary and that the brain produces consciousness. I think we have to revise our understanding of consciousness. Without more funding and more research, it's really difficult to verify, but I believe people's understanding is changing now. Thankfully, NDE experiences are taken slightly more seriously than they were 20 years ago. We still can't explain them, but we can't explain them away either. These are important experiences and we have to ensure that patients who have them are fully supported in coming to understand them as well."

Dr Eben Alexander continues this theme, "There's absolutely been a change in attitudes, which is very positive and affirming. There's been a huge uptick in peer-reviewed literature on NDEs since around 2013 and, I would say, a tremendous upsurge in scientific interest.

A huge body of scientific evidence points to consciousness that is independent of the brain. This emerging scientific model, in many ways, is such a gift. It really opens up our ability to see our relationship with each other and with the Universe in a positive fashion. In many ways, that is a reality the world is coming to recognize, and certainly those involved in scientific studies of NDEs, OBEs and past-life memories in children."

Liminal Life Lessons

Taking notice of the accounts of NDE or OBE experiencers may help our understanding of the liminal stages between life and death. After all, these accounts are the closest thing we have to knowing categorically what actually happens when we die.

Until we have that fuller picture, what advice or techniques do our experts recommend to make us feel more at ease around our dying loved ones and around the natural fear of our own inevitable demise? How do we accept that liminality?

Expert Inspiration #One

In her role as a soul midwife, Felicity Warner urges relatives to try not to look at the machinery and to home in on their loved ones; to hold their hand and to talk to them, even if they're in hospital.

She says, "We all have a different idea about what a good death is for us, but universally, from my experience, a good death is where we have been able to talk to our loved ones. To be able to tell them what it is that we want, we need and we hope for, and to have chosen, if we can, where we would like to die. It's becoming more and more common that people say they would like to die at home or at a hospice. We can support people by having these deep conversations without feelings of awkwardness or fear, but being open, honest and authentic.

"And saying we're sorry for things is a big thing as well – you know, the forgiveness thing. Saying we love people is another one. And to realize that this is a really sacred time, but full of potential for healing. Although that sounds like a paradox when someone is dying, the potential here is for healing. It's to become whole again and also for everybody around them to be able to partake in the death, almost as a healing journey for all of them. I believe that when you have that coming together, it really does change the experience of death enormously."

Expert Inspiration #Two

Penny Sartori's advice for those who experience an NDE is to get in touch with a support group or an organization such as NDEUK, which helps people to understand their experience. NDEUK offers regular online events to answer questions for people who are still coming to terms with what they experienced. Sartori believes it can be helpful to talk to other NDE experiencers and to realize that, even if your experience in uncommon, there will still be others who have undergone something similar.

"In the research, all of the people who have this experience come to the realization that we're all one; we're all part of this great consciousness. So, what we do to others, ultimately, we're doing to ourselves. When they have a life review, they can see how they've interacted with other people and how it feels to be in their shoes. They know what it's like to be on the receiving end of their own actions, both good and bad, and they can see the ripple effects of that down the line as well. The ultimate message is to treat others as you would wish to be treated yourself. That's at the heart of all the wisdom traditions, and if we could all live by that, wouldn't the world be totally different."

Expert Inspiration #Three

Dr Eben Alexander is clear that there are lessons to be learned about consciousness generally from NDEs, and that the individuals who have an NDE take on board specific life-changing lessons. He says, "I would say that the benefit is becoming more whole, becoming more of who we came here to be, both as individuals and as sentient life writ large throughout the entire planet, throughout the cosmos. For the individual, that often translates into something as simple as that physical, mental, emotional healing and wholeness are ultimately spiritual in nature. Ultimately, it affects how we live our lives: kindness, compassion, forgiveness and – the golden rule – treat others as you would like to be treated; that's written into the life review of Near Death Experiences going back thousands of years. In the life review, you relive various teaching points of your life, but often from the perspective of those around you who were affected by your actions, and even your thoughts. The life review is a beautiful example of how the boundaries of self that we see as so solid when we think about living our lives in these bodies are not so solid at all; that in fact, we're sharing the dream of the one mind.

"From the beginning, after my NDE, I often said that the biggest, most powerful lessons from the NDE community for the world are not what happens when you die, but far more critically, 'How do I live this life every day in my understanding of self, and self interacting with the Universe and with others?' That's where the NDE lessons are so powerful, to help us really mature and come into a much less ego-driven, but far more responsible and higher soul-driven sentient being. That's where the money is for this kind of NDE thing: it's to help the world grow up."

My Chapter Take-aways

- Undoubtedly, it can be hard to reverse the effects of death anxiety induced by living in a Western 'death-denying' culture, but by investigating different cultural beliefs surrounding death and death rites, especially those espoused by 'death-affirming' societies, it can help us to bring a different perspective to our fears.

- Spend more time around elderly relatives and loved ones and don't be afraid to talk to them about their beliefs and, if appropriate, their wishes when it comes to dying. It can be beneficial for you both and may be a comfort to you when the inevitable happens. My darling mum died during the pandemic aged 99. Remarkably, she did not fear death and we spoke openly about her belief in an afterlife. Sad though it was when she passed, and I still miss her, knowing her views helped me at the time.
- Back in the 1980s, Professor Kenneth Ring taught a class at the University of Connecticut on Near Death Experiences, and he found that his students were changed in much the same way as people who've had the NDE, simply by learning about them. I can certainly confirm that researching NDEs for this book has made me re-evaluate and live my life differently. If this topic interests you, and you want a glimpse into what it's like to experience a trip into the liminal space between life and death, try reading more of the NDE and OBE literature. (There are suggestions at the end of this book).

3

OPENING THE DOORS OF PERCEPTION

My research into the dying process, and more specifically NDEs and OBEs, raised serious questions about consciousness and our current understanding of it. I had already planned to consider the liminal spaces that lie at the outer edges of our consciousness, those faculties and abilities that we so rarely tap into, but there were some fundamental issues around the very nature of our accepted view of consciousness as raised by the NDE experts that warranted further discussion.

From her research into NDEs, Penny Sartori had come to her own conclusions about what an NDE might be. She says, "It seems to be a heightened state of consciousness. To all intents and purposes, it might be that the patient is flatlined at that particular point, their heart is not beating so their brain is not receiving oxygen, so they should not be having any conscious experience at all. But what they're reporting is a heightened state of reality. The thing is, all sensory input stops at that point as well. So, to me, it's more logical that consciousness is primary and that the brain does not produce consciousness."

Neurosurgeon and NDE experiencer Dr Eben Alexander describes the debate about where consciousness resides by saying, "If you keep it simple, you could just say consciousness is that very straightforward awareness of existence. All sentient beings are aware of our existing, and consciousness is nothing more magical than that self-awareness. Yet, to explain it, you have to go really, really deep.

"The empirical evidence for phenomena such as Near Death Experiences and especially the long work on past-life memories in children suggesting reincarnation, are some of the strongest lines of evidence in this whole discussion about the primacy of mind vs. eternity of soul. A more sensible alternative is seeing the one universe we live in, but with consciousness as fundamental and primary in that universe."

I turned to Anthony Peake, a writer about the borderline areas of consciousness, his latest book being *Cheating the Ferryman: The revolutionary science of life after death*, the sequel to his bestselling, *Is There Life After Death?* and offered him the challenge of giving a definition of consciousness. He patiently made a valiant and lengthy stab at helping me to understand. Starting with some background, he explains, "This is the great mystery of modern science. In 1994, at a conference about consciousness at the University of Arizona, a young Australian philosopher called David Chalmers stood up and pointed out that the soft problem of consciousness is how the brain works, how the neurochemicals work together, how the areas of the brain work together, all of which is solvable, but that science needs to address the hard problem, which is how does inanimate matter, chemicals reacting with electricity within the brain, create a self-aware consciousness that has a history, a background, memories, anticipations and everything else? And we're not even at first base in understanding this. We are no further down the route of understanding how something that is non-physical, i.e., thought and awareness and consciousness, can create movement within the body. How do I move my hand? What is the motive, the force that creates that? And this is the huge mystery.

"In the final analysis, everything we perceive is given to us by our awareness; there is nothing else other than I am something perceiving something. So, the question is much deeper. At the prime level, consciousness is the prime substance and from consciousness comes everything."

The scientists kept telling me to dive deeper, yet I was already in over my head. This was a hard concept to get my mind around. I asked Anthony Peake to explain it to me in terms of a Near Death Experience, since I felt I had a loose grasp on this at least.

He obliged, saying, "I'd argue that in an NDE, the brain starts to function differently. The brain is like a radio that picks up a signal, and the signal is out there. It's not inside our bodies. When someone has an NDE, they suddenly find themselves out in the greater information field, which means they can perceive things outside of their body. There are reported cases of NDEs where they report back information that they couldn't possibly know. The only answer is that they were seeing things that they should not be able to see. Individuals who have flatlined seem to perceive things but that is not possible because the brain is non-functional – there is no processing going on in the brain. Yet, they're still seeing, they're still hearing, they're still feeling. So, there's something here that is telling us something extraordinary about consciousness. Consciousness is outside the brain."

If consciousness lay outside of us, I couldn't help wondering why it was not possible for all of us to perceive this liminal information field at all times?

Peake pointed me in the direction of the writings of people such as philosophers Henri Bergson and CD Broad, and author Aldous Huxley, all of whom argue that the brain is a reducing valve. Thankfully, he also summarized their viewpoints, with which he concurs, saying, "Ordinarily, the brain works in a certain way and keeps reality steady. It gives you the reality that you need in order to function within the simulation. Under certain extreme circumstances or under the influence of certain chemical substances, that gets broken down and the brain's ability is stopped. The doors of perception are open and consciousness is then allowed to perceive the wider universe that ordinarily we are denied. And that's what happens when somebody has an NDE. This is what happens when somebody has an Out of Body Experience. It suddenly opens the doors of perception to the person to start perceiving a greater reality. It's extraordinary."

Penny Sartori has also come to a similar conclusion. She says, "To me, it's logical that consciousness is primary.

I think the brain acts like a filter. It screens out this consciousness that's around us all the time, but there are times when that filter action becomes dysfunctional or inactive. In an NDE, when there's no sensory input, there's nothing else to distract you, you're just there in this pure consciousness."

A New Paradigm Shift

At this point, a viewpoint from a non-scientist might be helpful. The obvious choice for a more philosophical view was writer and former investigative journalist, Daniel Pinchbeck, author of *Notes from the Edge Times.* He put our current world view of consciousness into perspective for me, saying, "With Christianity, there came a demonization of direct mystical experience. Missionary knowledge was at the beginning of the scientific revolution, which prioritized the left brain or the rational and masculine aspects of the psyche, and required a demonization of the right brain or intuitive visionary aspects of the psyche. So, that led to the witch hunts, the attacks on indigenous spiritual practitioners, at least while we were practising colonialism. At that time, it was a whole new mindset and ideology that demonized visionary experience.

"At the cutting edge of science, there are some areas that are trying to change that but, even so, we're still in the inertia of the old scientific, materialist paradigm, even though quantum physics has actually outmoded that view.

You still have prominent atheists who say that any kind of psychic or paranormal experience is totally invalid – it couldn't exist because the mind is just embedded in the physical hardware of the brain. So, there is still a paradigm war."

Although he believes this area of research needs more people doing research in the subject to move it forward, Anthony Peake also admits that a new breed of scientists is advancing the consciousness research and coming up with new ideas. Some scientists, and he names Max Tegmark at MIT and Vlatko Vadrel at the University of Singapore among them, are looking for new explanations in the realm of digital information and quantum physics. And quantum physics has shown objectively, particularly by what's known as 'the observer effect', that consciousness is essential to the chosen quantum state of an observed object, in the case of the most well-known piece of research on the behaviour of sub-atomic particles.

Dr Eben Alexander has seen a sea-change in the science community too. He feels that not only is the scientific world waking up to the new possibilities surrounding the non-local, liminal nature of consciousness, but that the public are now more interested too: "The challenge of COVID, with all the global death, the polarization it's brought to society, certainly in the US, and its unnerving effects should allow people to open up to a deeper interpretation of the data concerning their relationship with the Universe, and really their purpose for existence. The world just seems to be so energized by this polarizing energy and the conflict in our society that it doesn't leave a lot of room for that kind of introspection and allowing for a grander view of our relationship with the Universe.

"Yet, from my point of view, there's already been tremendous progress in the last decade or two, far beyond where we were before. I actually think that the revolution in coming to realize the primacy of consciousness and the unity that we share on a very deep level in a spiritual universe is a quiet revolution that sneaks up from beneath. Some of my main critics from eight and ten years ago are now realizing that this is the pathway forward, this is where the facts lie, and they are coming to accept this new model."

Why Explore Consciousness?

Although by now, I was starting to get a clearer understanding of the new science surrounding the liminal space that is consciousness, one question remained for me: why? Perhaps it had something to do with my journalist training, but I couldn't get beyond the elephant in the room which, for me, was why do you want to step over the threshold into these little explored areas of our minds? How does it benefit us individually or as a species?

Daniel Pinchbeck believes that, "Some people have very natural access to different states of consciousness; other people need help. We have to look at everything and its benefits to society. It's about exploration, you know. We have this consciousness, and therefore we have access to other dimensions of it. It's a natural part of us to seek, to explore those other aspects."

Pinchbeck also points out, "It's an innate human dispensation to want to explore these other dimensions or aspects of consciousness, just for curiosity, for self-development, for enlightenment, for healing others, even for power. There's a whole bunch of reasons, but throughout human history, we've been limited by our societies. Now we have scientists who are exploring this. The University of Virginia's Department of Perceptual Studies is looking at Near Death Experiences; Imperial College London is trying to understand the mechanics of psychedelic experience, or extraordinary human experience."

Science, it seems, is now lending credence and support to the age-old beliefs and views of the spiritual wisdom traditions. Nonetheless, Anthony Peake prefers to fall back on science, explaining that the Universe is a far stranger place than we can ever imagine, but that it works within the science. He says, "The new science is starting to realize that we have to understand consciousness, and by understanding consciousness, we will understand a great deal more about the Universe and how the Universe functions." Yet, he agrees with Pinchbeck that scientists like him do the research because they have an overriding need to understand what really is happening. "Some of us find the current materialist view unsatisfactory. We need to know more – what is the human condition and why? Most people are happy to live their lives without ever thinking about these things, and you can function perfectly well like that. But then, there is that dark night of the soul when you wake in the middle of the night and go, 'Is this it? Is this all I am? I'm just the link in a genetic chain? I'm just something that's perceived something for an infinitesimally small amount of time in the overall time of the Universe, and then I cease to exist again. Or is there more? And if there's more, what is there?' The greatest mysteries have to be, why am I here? What is the purpose of my life? Can I make life better? As human beings, it's what we want to do; we want to understand."

Aids to Exploring Consciousness

Steve Taylor is a senior lecturer in psychology at Leeds Beckett University and former chair of the Transpersonal Psychology section of the British Psychological Society. His latest book, *Extraordinary Awakenings: From Trauma to Transformation* is a collection of stories from those who discover a higher consciousness under extreme circumstances. He is the author of many other bestselling books on psychology and spirituality and his work has been described by Eckhart Tolle as "an important contribution to the shift in consciousness which is happening on our planet at present."

Steve says, "Everybody shares the same spiritual essence in terms of consciousness, so I think our own consciousness is an influx of the consciousness of the Universe itself. There is something inside us that is impersonal, which is fundamental and essential to the

Universe. We can touch into it in states of meditation. We can touch into it when we're in nature. When our minds become quieter. The moments of deep connection. It's always there. Often, our lives are too busy or our minds are too busy and we lose connection, we forget that it's there. We become so caught up in the ego mind, or too caught up in the activities of our lives, that we fall into a state of forgetfulness, but it's always there and it will always come back to us. In these moments of transformation, really what happens is that the ego breaks down and we become one with the essence of ideas again."

With the exception of those who are psychic or on a spiritual path of enlightenment and seeking to tap into a greater consciousness, since most of us are distracted by our busy lives, the most likely path to an increased interest in consciousness is if someone has a traumatic life event such as an NDE or OBE.

I ask Anthony Peake about catalysts for an interest in consciousness for those who are not already in the scientific or spiritual worlds. He says, "It's usually when people are taken out of their comfort zone, because they have an extraordinary experience that they cannot explain, when they start to think about consciousness. They have a Near Death Experience or an Out of Body Experience, they lucid dream, they encounter entities, they encounter spirits or see a ghost, these kinds of things, then suddenly their worldview changes totally. The nice steady world suddenly starts to evaporate around them and they start to question. I know dozens of people who have had these experiences and suddenly everything changes, suddenly what they believe is real changes. I've only ever had one lucid dream, and it was extraordinary. It changed me completely and changed my worldview."

Within the realm of altered states of consciousness (ASCs), there are those that are naturally occurring, such as Near Death Experiences and Out of Body Experiences, and then there are the artificially created experiences, known as Raised Consciousness (RCs). These RC states are attained by the consumption of substances called entheogens, which can be man-made – such as LSD and dimethyltryptamine (DMT) – or naturally occurring plant-based substances, such as ayahuasca and psilocybin (magic mushroom). Those who have experienced altered states of consciousness via both routes report that there is no real differentiation between the two. The question then is, what is it about these substances and these experiences that can take you into an alternate reality or alternate perception, to pass beyond the veil?

Anthony Peake believes there are certain substances that override the brain's ability to act as a filter. He says, "There is a group of scientists now particularly interested in going back to the ayahuasca/DMT area of research, and it's not just general scientists but anthropologists as well who are highly interested in the traditional experience of altered states of consciousness, particularly shamanism and the way that with rhythmic dancing and taking entheogens, you can enter another reality, another liminal space as it were."

I could see there and then that I needed to take a closer look at entheogens and other techniques such as meditation that can help to tap into the liminal, to have access to a wider realm of consciousness than is normally available to us. Before I did so, I asked Anthony Peake one last question about those who naturally have an ability to see a broader consciousness than the rest of us. Do we all have that latent ability?

"I'll guarantee that you will have experienced an altered consciousness; it's when you're half asleep, half awake, and you'll see faces in profile, or you'll hear voices. It's known as hypnagogia (as you're falling asleep) and hypnopompia (as you're waking up), and again, it's when the doors of perception are being broken down.

"We normally see this tiny little bit of the Universe. We believe that there's nothing else other than the visual world we can see. Yet we see only a small part of the electromagnetic spectrum. There is this whole visual world out there that we cannot see. A bat sees by sound. It bounces sound off objects and creates a visual image in its mind. That visual image is nothing like the visual world that we have. Bees see in ultraviolet so a rose doesn't look anything like it looks to us, to a bee. So, who's right?

"What I think happens is that there is a spectrum, I call it the Huxleyan spectrum, and the further along it you are, the more the doors of perception are going to be opened for you. I argue that there are neurotypicals, normal people who see the world as everybody sees it. Then you start moving into those with migraine, where you see aura states or you see the world slightly differently. I have migraine and I see zigzag patterns and all kinds of weird things. Then you move into temporal lobe epilepsy (TLE) – people who experience TLE have extraordinary experiences. They can fall out of time, or see entities. A friend and colleague who has had TLE all his life sees completely different worlds imposing themselves upon this one. Other fields on the spectrum include Charles Bonnet syndrome and types of autism, such as Loud World Syndrome (hyperacusis), where autistic children hear sounds that we don't hear, see things that we don't see. Then there are psychics, and you're getting broader and broader. Then you get into other areas such as Alzheimer's disease and dementia. As a person is coming toward the end of their life, their perception starts to get wider and wider. They start to have visions, or to see dead people. What's happening here, I believe, is that the doors of perception are opening."

The Consciousness Spectrum

The idea of a spectrum which, depending upon where you sit upon it, allows greater or lesser perception of a wider consciousness holds appeal for me and makes sense of why most of us are unable to tune in to this wider vision. It certainly goes some way toward explaining the amazing gifts of those with savant syndrome, many of whom have autism spectrum disorder (ASD). One of the most celebrated examples of the extraordinary abilities of someone with savant syndrome is the case of Stephen Wiltshire who, in 2009, took a 20-minute helicopter ride above New York City before being taken to the Pratt Institute in Brooklyn where he spent the next week producing a 19-foot long detailed, building-by-building rendition of that aerial view, correct in every detail. Other savants have exhibited the ability to:

- Memorize whole books with perfect recall of every word after simply glancing at the pages.
- Perform extraordinary mathematical calculations.
- Display musical genius, such as being able to expertly play an instrument on first picking it up.
- Speak multiple languages fluently.
- Measure exact distances visually without the aid of instruments.

Closer to home, what particularly grabbed my attention was the mention that people with dementia or Alzheimer's disease might also be on this spectrum and able to travel across the portal into a wider realm of consciousness. In 2003-2004, I witnessed my own father's descent into dementia at the end of his life. He experienced frightening episodes of what we then thought of as delusional fantasy. He often relived his distressing war experiences, and things that he had read in the newspaper or seen on the television became a reality for him in his mind and he was in the thick of it. My young sons at the time called these psychotic episodes, 'Poppa's Maisy Do's' and they passed quite quickly if we were sympathetic and played along, but they were extremely confusing and upsetting for us all. I found it intriguing that there might possibly be another explanation for these episodes other than the medical one.

Maggie La Tourelle is a psychotherapist, counsellor and author of the book and blog, both entitled *The Gift of Alzheimer's*. The book is an account of her mother's Alzheimer's journey and La Tourelle's perspective on it. It is also an excellent guide for those involved in the care of people with Alzheimer's disease. She explains that, "With Alzheimer's, the brain activity slows down, there's a loss of access to short term memory, past and future move into the present and you lose your sense of self and ego. I think that's the key thing. If you are without an ego in the present, you are potentially in a transcendental state, in which people have love, enlightened thoughts, extrasensory perception and pre-cognition. In her transcendent state, my mother was in another dimension that was out of space and time. That's my feeling."

The overriding message that La Tourelle took from her shared experience of her mother's passing is something that her mother said to her: "Love is the gateway between two worlds," and she also told her daughter that she had experienced, "the stillness of deep love" on the other side.

Liminal Life Lessons

It seems that institutional science would still have us believe that consciousness is seated in the brain, whereas the experts that I have spoken to support a paradigm shift in thinking that points toward a greater consciousness, an information field outside of us, if you will, that we can tap into.

Whichever stance you favour, science does not appear to be able to categorically explain consciousness one way or the other. It strikes me that if centuries of study of the function of the brain in neuroscience still can't locate where our memories are stored in the brain, then perhaps we should be open to exploring a nonlocal consciousness. Since the scientific jury is still out, I guess each of us has to make up our own minds on this thorny issue. What is clear to me is that the major questions that an interest in consciousness throws up – who am I? How do I relate to others and to the outside world? – are all worth giving greater consideration.

While you and I might ponder these big issues from the comfort of our armchair or maybe while we wander in the majesty of nature, there are many seekers who are actively using tools such as meditation, shamanic practices, hypnosis and the ingestion of plant medicines or synthetic entheogens to aid their passage across the threshold into an altered consciousness. We'll take a look at their experiences in the next chapter, but I want to finish with some practical advice and food for thought from our experts on consciousness.

Expert Inspiration #One

Dr Eben Alexander finds the materialist scientific thinking – i.e., that chemical reactions and electron fluxes in the brain are totally responsible for all thoughts, attitudes and beliefs – a bleak, nihilistic view that denies us any free will or responsibility for our actions. He says, "The emerging scientific model in many ways is such a gift. It really opens up our ability to see our relationship with each other and the Universe in a positive fashion. In many ways, that is a reality that the world is coming to recognize and, certainly, those involved in scientific studies. I believe this new model is closer to the truth and it opens up a tremendous amount of optimism and freedom to help take this world in a positive direction.

"I would say that one of the deepest, most powerful lessons that comes out of this emerging science of consciousness is that we have a very deep and profound responsibility for our choices, because they matter. All of emerging reality depends in many ways on the kind of choices and beliefs and attitudes of sentient beings; we're kind of guiding emergent reality. To deny that sense of responsibility can be very damaging.

"Yet I believe world peace is very possible. We just have to have a shift in perspective and a different understanding of ourselves in our relationship to the world at large, and also our very purpose and meaning in life. All of it coalesces to allow us to grow into a position of maturity that will help save this planet and really save all our souls."

Expert Inspiration #Two

Penny Sartori says, "Personally, it makes far more sense to me that we're all part of this great consciousness. We're not bodies that create consciousness; it's not the brain that creates it. It's already there, it's primary and we're part of it. We're spiritual beings having a temporary human experience. When we die, we go back to that original consciousness. It's eternal, and we have different experiences of it in a human body. For me, that makes much more sense and it's a comfort."

Expert Inspiration #Three

Anthony Peake agrees wholeheartedly with Sartori that more research is needed into the mystery of consciousness, saying, "You've got to have people like us, pushing the boundaries, trying to understand what's going on." The lesson that he takes from his study of the subject is: "We are one consciousness experiencing itself subjectively. Human consciousness is a collective, we are one consciousness and we are individuated consciousness. There is a direct relationship between us and out there. To me, it's wonderful and it's liberating, and it makes me accept my life far better."

Expert Inspiration #Four

The positive that Daniel Pinchbeck believes we can take from experiences of liminal space and of a broader consciousness is, "I would say that these types of transcendent experiences add value to people's lives. In the case of Near Death Experiences for example, the evidence seems overwhelming that people feel more positive, more connected, their lives have more meaning and they feel that death isn't the end, after an NDE.

"Typically, you can look at the John Hopkins study on psilocybin and consciousness. People who'd had a psychedelic experience for the first time felt that they had a permanence, or at least, very long-term positive shifts in their psychological evaluations, and more openness to new experience and so on.

"In the future, we'll see that consciousness is something that is innate in our human capacities, and we'll want to make it a central focus of the future of civilization."

Expert Inspiration #Five

After her own experience with her mother and then from her research, Maggie La Tourelle is confident that people with Alzheimer's spend time in another dimension and that, with understanding, their passing can be a more positive, conscious process. While remaining as calm and loving as possible, La Tourelle recommends the following way of relating to your loved one: "If they can talk, really listen. If they're telling you things, engage with them in their world. Don't try and pull them back into your world; and validate their experiences, even if they seem off the wall. You can say, 'That seems wonderful' or 'That seems difficult for you.' And if you do that with a loving presence, I really think the rest will just happen. It's very simple. I call it LEV with LP – Listen, Engage, Validate, and do it with a Loving Presence. You don't need to have any spiritual awareness to do that. And, when somebody is disturbed or remembering difficult times, use the statement, 'Everybody does the best they can at the time. If they could have done anything better, they would have done.' That's a very forgiving position to take and it's something that everybody can learn. With these tools, there is a process of building trust; and the more trust there is, the more they will speak to you. In that way, Alzheimer's provides an opportunity for conscious dying."

My Chapter Take-aways

- Consciousness is a vast and fascinating subject and our understanding of it is evolving all the time. If it interests you, I suggest that you delve into consciousness more deeply by reading up on the subject, watching podcasts or attending a webinar or workshop. Some of the leading lights in the field include Rupert Sheldrake, Gregg Braden, Joe Dispenza, Bruce Lipton, Rupert Spira, Steve Taylor, David Hamilton, Eckhart Tolle and Abraham Hicks.

- You can come at the subject of consciousness from various angles – science, humanities, religion, spirituality or mysticism. Why not start your research from whatever perspective feels comfortable and then leap into the liminal and approach it from one of the other less comfortable perspectives for you? Personally, I am most drawn to the spiritual approach to higher consciousness but I am now starting to explore non-dualism through the prism of the world religions in their esoteric branches, and I have been impressed by the scientific approach of experts such as Bruce Lipton and Joe Dispenza.
- There is an annual event held in the UK and America called TCCHE (The Conference for Consciousness and Human Evolution). Pay it a visit if you want to find out more.
- All of these suggestions are passive, theoretical approaches to the subject of consciousness. In the next chapter, we look at tools and approaches for exploring the liminal edge realms of consciousness, and I will make some practical suggestions you might like to explore at the end of that chapter.

4

MIND-ALTERING PRACTICES AND SUBSTANCES

The entheogenic properties of plant medicines have been used for centuries in some tribal and shamanic traditions, not only as a way to commune with the spirits but also as part of a healing process. Our forebears relied heavily on tree and plant magic, and the local wisewoman would be called upon for her knowledge of the healing properties of local herbs and plants. We know that the botanical knowledge of these traditional peoples was broad, and it's worth remembering that they used pharmacologically active plants not just as medicine and hallucinogens, but also as a poison – the difference often being only a matter of dosage. In the past, wise women knew that the active principals of certain European hallucinogens – including belladonna (Atropa belladonna), henbane (Hyoscyamus niger), mandrake (Mandragora officinarum) and datura (Datura metel) – can be absorbed directly through the skin. It's now believed that medieval witches commonly rubbed specific areas of their bodies with hallucinogenic ointments to experience the feeling of flying, for example. Across the world, in south-western Mexico, the Aztecs were preparing a sacred decoction known at one time as ololiuqui, from the crushed seeds of the morning glory (Rivea corymbose). It is thought that it was taken to induce altered states of consciousness in healing rituals and religious ceremonies. We now know that this contained alkaloids closely related to LSD, a potent synthetic hallucinogen. Similar brews from local psychoactive plants were used by shamans across the world to assist in their shamanic journeying, a practice used to this day to help them to commune with the spirits and to find answers, information, healing, wisdom, knowledge and guidance.

There are modern-day pharmaceutical psychedelic equivalents to these ancient potions that were studied extensively by government-backed researchers in the mid-twentieth century, and which are currently receiving a resurgence in interest in scientific circles. In addition, ancient and modern practices and modalities are also used to help move us through the liminal gateway to an altered consciousness. My quest was to find out more about these substances and practices, and also to expand my understanding of the liminal spaces into which these tools help those who use them to travel.

My starting place was with the traditional shamanic approach to journeying and plant medicine, and who better to speak to than Chris Odle, who trained in the Mestizo shamanic tradition in Peru in 2004? Since then, he has been running La Medicina plant sanctuary in the high jungle of the Peruvian Amazon, offering retreats to help guests find lasting healing and transformation. He explains, "Ayahuasca and plant medicines can reveal unitive consciousness within us, breaking down the barriers between 'self' and 'other', something that helps many [guests] regain their sense of spiritual connection."

While Western users of plant entheogens are frequently seeking a connection to source or higher consciousness, the local Amazonian population takes a wider view of the benefits of plant medicines. They use the shamans' working relationship with the forces in the unseen world via entheogens such as ayahuasca for a multitude of reasons, ranging from curing illness and improving hunting skills to ritual ways in which to bond the community and for divination to guide the tribe or the individual. Odle tells me, "In terms of the broad picture of liminal spaces, in traditional cultures, the boundaries between secular and the sacred are much more porous. If you take an indigenous long house, a *maloca*, where the family would live, the sacred and the profane are all part of normal life, essentially in the same space. There's no real separation. The same space could be used for cooking, washing and preparing meals and later on, in the evening, it could be a ceremonial space. As societies have developed, those boundaries have become a lot more clearly defined.

"Similarly, in indigenous myth beliefs, the manifestation of spirit was much more porous too. So, when you died, you could become a spirit or an animal, or you could change temporarily into an animal during your lifetime... The boundaries between self and the ontological other were much more porous. This boundary became more defined as the modern mind developed. So, to put people into the liminal space, it now perhaps needs stronger rituals than before, because people are so detached from the spirit in their lives, however you define that."

In developed countries, the most well-known plant medicine used for putting people into that liminal space is ayahuasca – a psychoactive brew made using the leaves of the Psychotria viridis plant and the stalks of the Banisteriopsis caapi vine. It may also contain other ingredients. Yet, Odle stresses that this is only one of the thousands of medicinal plants that local healers use to treat people. Each healer has their own repertoire of *remedios* (remedies), calling on a living library of plant knowledge that has been built up among the community of healers over centuries, if not millennia.

Author Danu Forest has studied and practiced Celtic shamanism as part of her PhD studies in Celtic tradition. She believes that, historically, the UK would have had our own shaman using local plants and entheogens to heal people and to help them to move into a liminal state. She says, "There are schools of thought that suggest that psilocybin mushrooms were used ritually here once upon a time in the same way that ayahuasca and other psychotropic plants are used in other parts of the world. I don't see why not. It seems to me that these things were probably happening simultaneously around the world, so it would be odd if we didn't have an equivalent of some sort. We have psilocybin mushrooms and fly agaric toadstools, and they both have shamanic uses, but we've lost the lore around how to use them in a good therapeutic sense, and we've lost whatever rituals and framework there would have been around the taking of them.

"With all the privileges that have come with Western life, we have quite seriously pulled away from our roots and that connection. As a culture, we no longer identify these lands and our landscape with the ability to give us medicines or what we need to be whole. Yet, as a practitioner, I feel that the spirits are here for us as much as they ever were; they've never gone anywhere. Whether we call them gods, spirits or ancestors, whatever labels we put on them, they haven't left. The effects of Christianity, industrialization and technology all change, but waiting there at the other end of the line, the tool is still there. We still have, growing all around us, plants that can be of support in all sorts of ways, medicinally and psychologically, let alone spiritually. It's quite incredible."

Healing with Spirit

Danu Forest is helping people to learn to work with the spirit presences of our own landscape using Celtic shamanistic techniques and ceremony, and offering opportunities to explore the traditions and liminal spaces of the British Isles and Ireland, but she is almost a lone voice, while those traditions are still strong in the Amazon. Yet even in a thriving shamanic locality such as Peru, there is one practice that is under threat. Known as the *dieta*, it is a way to prepare the body for the sacred space of the plant medicine and ceremony. Modern Peruvians do not want to adopt the stringent principles of abstinence but these practices have their roots in spiritual purification, which is important. Chris Odle says, "From the perspective of Amazonian shamanism, the spiritual aspect of disease is viewed as the root cause and is thus more important than the purely physical. The *dieta* is a core principle and involves isolation, sexual abstinence and a restricted simple diet to purify and open the body/spirit to the energies of the plants you are consuming so they can work within you. You could say you're providing a liminal space in the body for the plants to enter.

"The cause of illness, certainly in Amazonian shamanism, was either breaking food taboos, for example, over-consumption of certain game-animals or fish in a particular season, or serious illness was often considered witchcraft from another tribe. In both cases, the shaman was called upon to mediate and to negotiate with the ontological other to restore balance. The Western idea that there's the emotional self and the psychological self, the fragmentation of the psyche, that just didn't exist for the early tribes. For them, all illness was spiritual in some sense."

While indigenous peoples might seek out the village shaman for wisdom as well as for healing, I wondered what motivated the Western visitors who come for ayahuasca journeys, given our very different understanding of illness and the possibilities that lie in the liminal states of altered consciousness? According to those I met, some people use retreats to deal with emotional issues or to address addiction problems, but it seems that the majority are looking for transformation in their lives and greater connection.

Someone who came to ayahuasca and plant medicines by a less conventional route is documentary maker, author and explorer Bruce Parry, star of the BBC documentary series *Tribe* and then *Amazon with Bruce Parry*. He told me, "I started out very much in the Western scientific materialist dogma paradigm. I was a former British Royal Marine, a Christian – I was of the institution." It was after leaving the forces that Parry was first tempted into trying a magic mushroom by a girlfriend. He continues, "That set me off on a spiritual journey, but that was just an opening. It was years later that I started on the *Tribe* series, and the first episode I filmed was a three-day initiation with a group called the Babongo in the Congo, where I did this hallucinogen called iboga. Although I did a fair bit of reading beforehand, I'd never done anything like it before and it was another huge step in my awakening. I had these universal consciousness kind of experiences, extraordinary empathic visions. I saw deities, all the sort of stuff that you can get from these deep medicine journeys, and yet I always maintained a subtly rational mind about it all.

"Later, I did a series called *Amazon with Bruce Parry*, where I took ayahuasca a few times and I continued to do ayahuasca journeys around the world. Ultimately, I went on a progressive journey of stepping stones, and started slowly absorbing a different type of belief system and a different relationship with myself; there was a lot of healing, which was vital. Alongside that, as I was lucky enough to be doing it with tribal people, there was also a deeper relationship with nature, which I enjoyed, because of their ancestral nature-related explanation to it."

Parry feels that while we have efficient medicines in our hospitals for physical ailments, when it comes to the mind, we don't have the same toolkit as the indigenous tribes whose plants can be helpful for problems of the psyche too. He says, "Ayahuasca, and similarly iboga to my mind, allows you to revisit trauma. Often, you'll go into sleep mode, have a vision of a moment in time that you might even have forgotten about, and you'll relive that experience where you were traumatized, but you will be able to see it from the perspective of a more mature and more compassionate being. Then, you have an opportunity to reroute the neural pathway to the amygdala of panic, shock or protection, or whatever was being reinforced, and therefore allow for a different perspective on that thing.

"Alongside that, because a lot of these traumas are stored in the stomach, you get a shifting and with that, possibly vomiting. It's a movement of the locked, stored energy that is located there. This is a very visceral experience: you relive something, you see it and you often then literally release it. It's very powerful, because you have an opportunity to behave differently. When faced with what would have been an unconscious behaviour, you can now act more harmoniously toward that, which is so vital for us today. We need that so much."

What Role does a Shaman Play?

Firstly, it's worth mentioning that 'shaman' is the word that has come into common parlance in the West to cover a wide range of traditional healers and plant medicine practitioners, but it is not a word that is found in the Amazon. There, you are more likely to hear the name *vegetalista* – someone who works with plants, an *ayahuascero* who works specifically with ayahuasca, or a *curandero* – a healer. But, since 'shaman' is such a readily understood catch-all in the West, I'll continue to use it for the purposes of this book.

It would seem that the role of the shaman ranges from that of an enabler who holds the space while you partake, to someone who performs rituals and directs the ceremony. In the tradition in which Odle trained, the shaman favours the former. He says, "When someone is ingesting the powerful plant medicine, there's sacred space in the *maloca*, but there is very little ritual in terms of saying prayer. The bottles are sung to, and individual doses are poured and sung to before they're served. The singing is important because that opens up a liminal space through the medicine songs as well as through the medicine."

Bruce Parry has experienced both styles, saying, "I've drunk with many shamans. In the ayahuasca realm itself, some are good in that they offer the plant, the medicine itself, and then step out of the way, maybe offering some music or song, but they don't interfere at all with your own personal journey. Others may hark up halfway through the ceremony, giving prayers and, although they're all beautiful, there's a lot of that person involved. And that's the beginning of a mediation. It's the same with the pulpit and all that stuff – it's about people getting in the way of your own direct connection. This goes on in the jungle as well as in the church. Power is at play and a shaman can have a very difficult job of not abusing that power, basically."

This leads Parry to talk about his most recent project, living with the Pirahã, an indigenous tribe from the Amazonas region of Brazil who still live an egalitarian lifestyle and who feature in his film, *TAWAI: A voice from the forest*. (*Tawai* is a word the nomadic hunter gatherers of Borneo use to describe the connection they feel to their forest home.) He says, "There was a time when we all had our own direct connection with the divine. I've experienced places where nearly everyone has their own direct connection and this guides them. The Pirahã in Brazil, who basically have no future and past tense to their language and are so present that just by going into the forest, they're able to connect with these entities. I asked them, 'How do these entities communicate with you?', and they said, 'Through our heart and then into our mind and then they guide us.' Whether this is a primitive intuition that's coming from the inside, or whether it really is tapping into a universal consciousness, I don't think we'll ever know, but it felt to me like it was a wise guidance that had deep ecological wisdom at its heart.

"My understanding is that we all once had our own direct connection, and we didn't need intermediaries when we were much more present, in the moment and less cluttered. So, the shamanic culture probably came about like all religious spiritual traditions, as a way of taking us back to something that we already once knew."

Seeking Connection via Other Routes

With or without the mediation of a shaman, the plant medicines can be considered a powerful tool to aid our connection and to help us to traverse more easily into the liminal space at the outer edges of our consciousness. The aim is to increase connection so it becomes always present, whatever you are doing in your life. As Chris Odle points out, "If you're connected within yourself, you're always in the liminal; you're always connected to source. Whether you're doing ayahuasca ceremonies, meditating or whatever your practice, you're keeping that connection going and hopefully deepening it, and it informs how you live."

From a mental health perspective, it's known that, when over-activated, the default mode network (DMN) in the brain (the network of interacting brain regions active when a person is not focussed on the outside world) is where your ego and all the negative self-talk resides. It's also acknowledged that depression and anxiety are more prevalent in people who have very active default mode networks.

The concept that psychedelics work by disrupting the DMN of the brain is widely accepted. The same principle applies to what might be considered milder tools and practices, ranging from mindfulness and meditation through to ritual and hypnosis – they are all ways to 'turn off' the DMN and allow you to use other parts of the brain. It was time to turn my attention to these other routes to greater connection.

Odle cites drumming as one example of ritual practice, "If you actually listen to shamanic drumming – I think it's 140 beats per minute – it's quite remarkable. Most people will be able to go into a visionary state."

Celtic shaman Danu Forest agrees. She says, "Drums are a powerful tool to help gain altered states of consciousness and awareness. In the Celtic traditions, we don't have much evidence for the use of drums early on – it's a later addition – but it's the best tool to access those states in many ways. We do have things like seeking visions by the side of rivers, where you can get lost in the white noise of the water. There's lots of examples of shaking bells – again, that kind of rhythmical white noise in the background. Silver bells or a silver branch appear in traditional stories to lull people to sleep where they encounter the other world. The sound of the wind in the trees and birdsong are also natural sounds traditionally used as a way to achieve altered states of awareness, but they are more subtle than the drum, which is still the best tool."

Some years ago, Bruce Parry experienced a Vipassana retreat. Vipassana, which means 'to see things as they really are', is one of India's most ancient techniques of meditation. It is a way of self-transformation through self-observation and focuses on the deep interconnection between mind and body. He says of the experience, "It's possible to have a similar type of experience, it's just a different way of getting there. Also, the narrative that supports the experience is different."

After his NDE, Dr Eben Alexander admits that he spent at least two years reading and researching consciousness, but soon came to realize that to understand it, you had to experience it. So, he looked for different meditation techniques to take him within. He says, "I now use sacred acoustics, that is differential frequency brainwave entrainment, to meditate for an hour or two a day. I've been doing that for more than a decade now and I've found it to be profoundly important in my own understanding. It helps me not only to recover the content of my NDE, but to actually re-engage actively with the denizens and spirit guides and everything else that I first encountered, in some flavour, in my NDE.

"With a powerful tool like Binaural Beat Brainwave Entrainment (BBBE), which puts a pure tone in one ear and a slightly different tone in the other, say 100 hertz in one and 104 hertz in the other, you get the 4 hertz wavering signal that interacts with the lower brainstem, which is a very ancient circuit. At workshops, I've heard plenty of stories of people who have had profound spiritual experiences – encountering souls of departed loved ones, having great insight – just many calming and beautiful effects. Out of Body Experiences can be enhanced by BBBE and they're very beneficial in helping people explore deeply in the conscious realm. You don't have to have an NDE to begin to assimilate and access that grander sense of conscious awareness; you can do it through meditation, or spontaneous epiphanies, prayer and the many other ways of going within."

Psychologist Dr Mike Dow has a post-doctoral education in clinical hypnosis and is the *New York Times* bestselling author of *Your Subconscious Brain Can Change Your Life* among other books. He tells me, "Hypnosis can offer a light form of the sort of altered or non-ordinary state of consciousness that you have with psychedelics. So, I created a hypnosis meditation track so that, if you've never experienced a psychedelic, you can actually just touch what it feels like. Obviously, psychedelics can take you much, much deeper, but you can have that sort of experience in light forms in everyday ways. For example, at Catholic mass, why do they have incense? And why does it swing back and forth? It's not dissimilar to when we train in clinical hypnosis and some of the methods we use, like staring at something that's swaying back and forth, like the pocket watch, right? It creates these altered states, and certainly in many religious traditions there's chanting and incense – all these things that we've used throughout the generations – is it maybe part of what we need as our world becomes increasingly secular? Is this the missing piece?

"I'm not here to tell people to be religious or not, but I certainly think that we've got to make room for and cultivate this liminal space, this transitional spiritual sense of awe, wonder and connectivity as necessary parts of the human experience. You can get it in the temple, at mass, in a meditation group, under hypnosis or using psychedelics, but I do think it's part of ourselves. It's alternating between the *doing* mind and the *being* mind, which they talk about a lot in mindfulness training, and I think psychedelics are the ultimate manifestation of the being. And not just being within the physical body of yourself, but a larger being of oneness."

The Science Behind the Practices

I understood that there was hard scientific evidence behind the effects of psychedelic drugs and that a lot was known about the constituent active ingredients of plant medicines and drugs, but was there any science behind the effects of other practices that lead us to an altered awareness?

Dr Mike Dow offered an explanation. "These spiritual practices are simply a way to facilitate the shift from sympathetic to parasympathetic nervous system activation: moving from 'fight or flight' to 'rest and digest'. We live in these chronic states of stress, we're in fight or flight all the time. As we know, most doctor's visits are stress-related – it's the grand activator of conditions that are already present, such as migraines or MS. What conditions are not made worse by stress? We have to slowly heal from constantly living in that stress state. People view it as optional but it's absolutely necessary for us to do so.

"In the modern world, we exploit sensation-seeking and reward-seeking neurotransmitters such as adrenaline and dopamine without doing any of the work. Take our phones – we get a little hit of dopamine every time there's a message or a 'like' on social media, and we're chasing that rush all the time. Connecting that to these other states, these transitional liminal states, these non-ordinary states of consciousness, you are moving away from this dopamine sensation-seeking and you're actually transitioning yourself to not just other parts of the brain, but I think also different neurotransmitters. These other neurotransmitters like oxytocin and vasopressin, which really bond us and connect us, and serotonin – feeling okay and present or GABA – feeling calm, easy and peaceful, are more strongly correlated with these altered states. In our society as a whole, we need more of these downers and probably less adrenaline and dopamine."

In other research studies, there is now data that shows that mindfulness meditation increases thickness in the prefrontal cortex and parietal lobes, both linked to attention control, while compassion-based meditation showed increases in the limbic system, which processes emotions, and the anterior insula, which helps bring emotions into conscious awareness.

Dr Eben Alexander is also knowledgeable on entheogens. He tells me of some fascinating research on this very subject. "If you use functional MRI scans or, more recently, Magnetoencephalography to look at neural activity – the activity of brain cells that are responsible for thoughts and emotions – you find that under the influence of something like psilocybin, the brain goes dark. The neural processing shuts off. The default mode network falls apart and disambiguates. Robin Carhart-Harris of Imperial College London also assessed the kind of transcendental profundity of the experience that someone had while on psilocybin, using the visual analogue scale (a line with one end meaning no transcendence and the other end meaning the deepest transcendence imaginable), and they found that in the people whose brain went the darkest, their experience was the broadest.

"This was a beautiful example, which rang true for me, having had my neocortex inactivated. More recent scientific papers include work from South America looking at DMT (Dimethyltryptamine), an active principle from ayahuasca plants, and more recent ones on LSD, the most powerful serotonin two-way entheogen, and all find the same thing: the brain goes dark, and the only realistic interpretation of that data is that there is no neuronal population at all that is supporting any of the phenomenal activity that people are witnessing.

"The first important point is that the scientific data shows the brain goes dark on these plant medicines. The second important point is that some investigators, for example at John Hopkins and UCLA in the US, have started using entheogens to treat addictions like alcoholism and opioid abuse, and to alleviate debilitating fear of death in terminal cancer patients."

So, I had my answer. There is plenty of scientific data explaining the neurological changes in the brain brought about by entheogens and by meditative practices, but as Dr Dow points out, that is only half the picture. The data does not fully explain the benefits of crossing into the liminal and exploring an altered consciousness. I ask him whether his medical training and his scientific understanding of the neural pathways and transmitters that explain so much of our behaviour ever conflicted with his personal experience of consciousness. He says, "I've thought about your question a lot and just because you understand it medically or structurally or from a neurotransmitter point of view, it's not the same thing as creating it. I can tell you that I've had experiences in my hypnosis, in psychedelic-assisted psychotherapy sessions, and just in my life when I've felt profound, deep love. In psychedelic research, we talk a lot about this noetic quality – not having the words to explain something away, but just this feeling of knowing.

"One of my favourite pieces of an interview from a participant in the John Hopkins psilocybin-assisted psychotherapy study was an atheist who said that it felt as though she was 'bathed in God's love.' And they said, 'but you're an atheist?' and she said, 'I know, but that's the only way I can describe it.' To have that experience, even for somebody who identifies as atheist, is incredible. It didn't change her religious belief, but certainly the experience of 'being bathed in God's love' changed her – and probably changed her forever, as my experience has for me. My belief comes from this deep knowing and experiencing.

It feels like the ultimate truth to me and that's why I have this greater understanding that is extremely spiritual. I do believe in things that can't be explained away by science."

However, he also concedes that it can be valuable to have modern technology, such as MRI scans, and better techniques that offer us some evidence. He says, "So many personality types need that. They need the scientific explanation and the evidence. So, yes, there are these real effects that we can study that hopefully will motivate people."

Dr Alexander draws a close to the science debate by telling me that he believes that, in particular, study of the clinical use of psychedelics in treating addiction and phobias is very important. However, he adds, "I've had personal experience with some of the psychedelics, in the scientific sense, to compare with my NDE and that specifically includes experience with 5-Methoxy-N, the most powerful form of that entheogen available, and I can tell you that it was like looking through a tiny keyhole into what I believe is the same kind of space for my NDE to happen, but the NDE is a broad panoramic penthouse suite view of that spiritual realm that the psychedelics cannot even remotely approach."

Therapeutic Uses

Dr Eben Alexander mentioned the addiction work using psychedelics, and quite by chance I learned through our conversations that Dr Dow was working at the cutting edge of this new form of treatment, in his case specializing in treating depression. He was eager to explain it to me, as he is fully convinced of its value in the treatment of both addiction and depression.

He says, "One of the best uses of psychedelics is for the treatment of addiction. It's interesting because it can sort of rewire and reset the brain in a way that is more effective than any other treatment we have. So, we're not trading a lesser evil, such as methadone, we are actually using something that increases neurogenesis, that increases neuroplasticity, connecting the brain."

Focussing on the more noetic, liminal aspects of entheogens and their uses, Dr Dow continues, "What's really interesting to me, and something that I've experienced in my own training with psychedelics because you actually have to take the drug to train in it, is the ego death. There's that wonderful quote that says 'the secret of life is to die before you die', which is the point of these liminal spaces. So whether you're using prayer, meditation, chanting or psychedelics, when you can have that ego death, and you realize that you can step out from some of the constructs that the ego creates, and you feel yourself as energy and matter that is no different from the matter or energy of other beings, it really does help people with these transitions and to live in them a little more.

"The letting go really allowed me to step outside and see something that was greater, and that for me was extremely healing. From a first-person point of view, I experientially understand why psychedelics are so healing for depression, trauma, and anxiety disorders."

Liminal Life Lessons

The liminal states that hold so much allure and promise for us are available to all but, apart from a few enlightened souls or those who have spontaneous Out of Body Experiences, most of us need to use techniques or tools to help us access those places.

These aids to altered consciousness range from rhythmic sounds such as shamanic drumming, gongs or crystal bowls, through healing modalities such as clinical hypnosis and binaural beats, to taking entheogens such as ayahuasca, psilocybin and other plant medicines or synthetics such as ketamine, 5-MeO-DMT or LSD.

The reasons to experiment with these techniques and substances are particular to each individual seeker, but the potential strikes me as far-reaching, most particularly in the field of healing and self-exploration. Let's see what final words of wisdom and advice our experts have for us:

Expert Inspiration #One
Dr Eben Alexander encourages us all to adopt a meditation practice to explore liminality more fully, saying, "I came to realize you can read books and study this stuff all you want, but ultimately, if you want to understand consciousness,

you need to explore it. After my NDE, I looked for different meditation techniques. I wanted to go within. I knew where the scientific data was leading, but I had to do it myself; I had to explore myself. You can tell people about all this till the cows come home, and you can offer them the models and tell the stories of people's experiences and all that helps, but if they're not going within themselves, then it's going to be a tougher battle to convince them."

Expert Inspiration #Two

La Medicina Ayahuasca retreat leader Chris Odle believes that "the mind is like a labyrinth to the unconscious, and once a lot of unconscious material is released and you become more conscious, beyond a certain point, you're always in a liminal state; surely that's the idea of all these practices? With plant medicine, the idea is that you get to the point where you don't need to take more plant medicines."

In his literature, he says, "We are both the ripple and the river. Ayahuasca and plant medicines can reveal unitive consciousness within us, breaking down the barriers between 'self' and 'other', something that helps many regain their sense of spiritual connection. When we get in touch with this deeper consciousness on a visceral level, the challenge is to then express it in our day-to-day lives. Rather than chasing peak experiences through more ceremonies with the danger of spiritually bypassing, we need to do whatever inner work is necessary to become more conscious of our heart, the place where the ripple dissolves into the river. When this happens, we live our life with a strong spirit, embodying the uniqueness of our connection to source."

He also sounds a cautionary note for anyone looking to experience an ayahuasca ceremony: "Plant medicines are powerful and so they're potentially dangerous as well. Without a strong ritual element and someone guiding it, it could be dangerous." So, make sure you research your experience carefully before committing. Another thing to consider in your choice is location. He says, "There are forces within the environment that add something to the experience, because you're working with the energies of the land, and that can be particularly true of plant medicine."

Finally, he stresses the importance of "humans gathering together and sharing liminal space as a way to express a deep yearning in all of us to reaffirm or connect to others. There's a beauty and a validity in that."

Expert Inspiration #Three

As well as offering us an opportunity to change our behaviours, Bruce Parry believes that plant medicines such as ayahuasca or iboga give us greater self-understanding. He says, "You get a chance to look at yourself and your behaviour and your actions. It's weird. It takes you to a space where you get to see yourself in a way that no shrink ever could, because you're seeing yourself not by someone else telling you, but you get to see who you are in that moment. That can be incredibly humbling as you can realize just how selfish or careless or aggressive or whatever it is that we are in our lives, and that opens a window into an understanding whereby you have an opportunity to make new decisions in your life. It gives you an insight, and this could be like the vision aspect of plant medicine, so you can readjust your behaviour.

"Finally, it invites you, and offers you in a very deep way, a feeling of connection. You can have this expansive letting go of the identification with the individual self and merge into what's beyond, which is the liminal space. That can be really beautiful, because it invites us to have an understanding that there's more to it than the physical form and what we think of as this life. In turn, that allows a different way of behaving in our life, because we can believe in something beyond. It can allow not only the joy of belief that there's something beyond, but also a reflection on how we behave now, because there is something that's going to come after. There's this extraordinary sense of interconnectedness with the Universe and all the different layers and elements that come with that."

Expert Inspiration #Four

Danu Forest believes the movement into a different consciousness of a shamanic vision quest is available to you wherever you may live, not just those in the Amazonian jungles. She says, "It would be wonderful if we all had access to a lovely roundhouse and some woods of our own, but essentially, if it's a case of making prayers to the spirits and the ancestors and making an offering, sitting in darkness to receive your vision, which is similar to shamanic practices all around the world, then actually, that's just as accessible in your sitting room in London as it is anywhere else. It's really empowering once people realize that.

"It really does work wherever you are. It's lovely to have that framework of being able to go up into the mountains, but it's not essential. It is about how well you can relate, how well you can access that liminal space within you, that little voice. It's what you bring that makes it work. It's your ability to relate to that wider 'all' that is the key skill, and that's something we all carry with us. We remove ourselves from it sometimes, but it's never actually removed from us."

Expert Inspiration #Five

Dr Mike Dow combines his medical training with a belief in a wider consciousness. He says, "I feel our physical bodies are vessels for our souls and our consciousness to live in for a time, and we shouldn't confuse the physical body with spirit, with consciousness. They are not one and the same."

Of his own experiences with hypnosis and psychedelics, he says, "I would say that the most profound lesson was one of love, and how my life is really an opportunity for love to work its magic. It's even hard to verbalize this, because so many of the lessons that I received in that liminal space were so ethereal, spiritual, tactile, visual, but they weren't everyday thoughts and feelings. The experience was pure love, and what love is all about. It left me feeling, 'Ah, that's the point of living.' It really transforms everything – the way you see yourself, the way you see the world. There's a lot of hopelessness and anger in the world right now, in terms of the pandemic and politics and global warming. I can see how the connectedness you get in those altered states can be a part of the shift in the healing that needs to take place. I think these liminal states are really necessary for the world and its healing."

My Chapter Take-aways

- If you want to experience the liminality of altered consciousness for yourself, you could start by attending a meditation class or retreat. I love it but I have friends who simply cannot lose themselves to the practice. Why not try a soundbath? At the very least it will create a deep state of relaxation within you, and some people experience their first taste of an altered consciousness via this route. There are other modalities and techniques, ranging from binaural beats to Tibetan singing bowls and shamanic drumming – I encourage you to do a bit of digging to discover which tool appeals.
- If all of the above sounds a bit too woo-woo for your taste, you could try a hypnosis session. That too can connect you to a liminal state. Hypnosis under the guidance of a trained professional could give you a taste of the more powerful altered consciousness experience induced by psychotropic plants and drugs. The state of hypnosis is a waking state of

awareness or consciousness in which your attention is detached from your immediate environment and, instead, it is absorbed by inner experiences. I have been hypnotized in the past and I would describe the feeling during hypnotherapy as being calm and extremely relaxed both mentally and physically, which allows you to focus on your inner voice. It is definitely a liminal experience, albeit milder than some of the other routes.

- I have to make a confession here. I have never experienced an ayahuasca ceremony or taken any entheogens. In my quest for a greater understanding of liminal space, I am toying with the idea of undergoing a ceremony, but since I routinely experience an altered awareness using the milder approach of meditation, I am still undecided. Should you be drawn to explore the liminal opportunities offered by a plant entheogen, then I would suggest that you carefully research the sort of ceremony that best suits your needs, and that you check testimonials and speak with the organizers before signing up. Plant medicines are powerful and you must be totally comfortable with the provider and the style of experience offered.

5

TAPPING INTO THE DIVINE

We know that those experimenting with tools to reach an altered consciousness often report a noetic, spiritual experience on their return from such states. In addition, research shows that 62 per cent of Americans hold New Age beliefs, such as the presence of spirit in trees or mountains. Meanwhile, in the UK, despite the decline of formalized religion, the country is a long way from being a nation of non-believers. According to a recent survey, three out of four Britons believe that spiritual forces have influence on the Earth and that there are things that science cannot explain. Moreover, over half of those surveyed (59 per cent) believe in the existence of some kind of spiritual being. More than one-third believe in God as "a universal life force", a similar number in spirits, and a quarter in angels. Some 12 per cent accepted the existence of "a higher spiritual being that cannot be called God". What of the liminal spaces that we enter when we search for spirituality and the divine using prayer or meditation?

For me, the big question for believers and non-believers alike centres on the liminal spaces that we enter when we search for spirituality and the divine using prayer or meditation.

Steve Taylor, in his latest book, *Extraordinary Awakenings,* chronicles the stories of people around the world who have experienced spontaneous spiritual awakenings. I asked him why he thought spirituality was becoming more popular at this particular time.

He says, "I often draw a parallel between individual transformation and collective transformation. It's quite common for people to undergo transformation when they're in situations of great turmoil. And now, collectively, we're in a situation of great turmoil, not just with the COVID pandemic, but the climate emergency and political instability – lots of different issues. I think our collective turmoil is having a transformational effect. Maybe that's why, if you look around the world, so many people are drawn to spirituality, so many people are looking for something beyond material values. Spiritual development is probably the most significant trend of our time.

"Twenty-five years ago, when I started getting interested in spirituality, it was like an underground movement. It wasn't easy to find books about spirituality, to talk to people about it or to find groups, but now it's changed a lot. It is almost like the flowering of a new kind of consciousness, as if a new level of human consciousness is slowly uncovering itself. There's even research showing that spiritual experiences have become more common over the past 30 years. In surveys, if you ask people, 'Have you ever had a spiritual experience in which you felt at one with the Universe?' almost twice as many people respond affirmatively than 25 years ago."

Neale Donald Walsch, author of the bestselling *Conversations with God* series of books that have sold many millions of copies worldwide and been translated into 37 languages, agrees. He says, "We live in an interesting time. We're in liminality. We're between what we thought we knew and what we don't know. Many people don't know which is which anymore."

I had been told by shamanic retreat owner Chris Odle that many modern Peruvians are turning their backs on the traditional shamanic approaches to medicine and ancient spiritual wisdom of their forebears, yet more and more Western seekers are travelling to the Amazon looking for a deeper experience. I asked him why he thought this might be. "It's to do with the stage of development that the country is at. The Western world has developed, a certain amount of comfort has been achieved, but it hasn't fulfilled the deeper spiritual needs. So, this whole wellbeing, spiritual, New Age movement has developed. If you take a country like Peru, for some of our workers, moving up from a dirt floor to a cement floor in their houses is a big thing, while in Lima, you've got a middle class who are making money, and they're doing yoga and exploring alternative therapies. So, if you look at the broader picture of how a country develops, how people have material lack and think they need more material comfort; then the country develops until they have material comfort and, in that process, old ways are often forgotten in the pursuit of material wealth. When that's achieved, there then comes a kind of connect to emptiness. Then there's a searching once again to rediscover their own spiritual roots, or through globalization to find some other kind of path."

What Are We Searching For?

Kindred Spirit magazine columnist and feature writer David Olliff has a first-class honours degree in Theology and describes himself as "Christian but not religious. I think I've become a sort of Christian occultist really. I'm a follower of Dion Fortune [a proponent of Christian mysticism]." During my time as his editor, I always knew I could rely on him for informative and thought-provoking articles on classic spiritual texts, among other things, so I turned to him to see if he could shed any light on what it means in this day and age to be spiritual.

"Spirituality is a very difficult space to talk about," he says. An inauspicious start, but Olliff was just warming to his subject. He continued, "It seems to me that people use spirituality as a way of developing on that journey to becoming their best selves. There is an inherent psychology built into that, but there is also a sense of a relationship to an Other. I think that's what the struggle of spirituality is – the relationship of the interior self in relation to the divine, which is other but also not other. That's one of the great problems of the liminal space you're talking about. We create this sense that there is maybe a God out there, but I feel it's more a sense of a God within, that is also out there, but there isn't a clear otherness.

"Liminal spaces are so difficult because it is our interiority, the interior itself, in relation to our experiences that are exterior and other. There is a microcosm and a macrocosm; the microcosm being the infinite world within, and who we are as individuals, and then the macrocosm being the whole of the rest of that eternal space. As physical manifest beings, we understand ourselves in terms of physical limits, so we're always at the boundary of something; we're always at the liminal of something. There is a full, almost limitless world interior to us, and there is another world that we have to somehow negotiate and engage within. We are experiencing things permanently at the shore, at the threshold."

Benefits of Being in the Sacred

It's still hard to understand what exactly happens when someone seeks enlightenment, when they welcome this liminality into their lives. What is it that they are pursuing? What are the benefits of being more spiritual? Steve Taylor comes up with something akin to a definition: "In purely psychological terms, a spiritual awakening is basically an expansion of awareness in lots of different ways: in perceptual terms, because the world becomes more real and beautiful; in subjective terms, because you journey deep into yourself and discover new things inside your own being; in social terms, because you connect more with other people and other living beings – you become more empathic and compassionate."

He continues, "Almost everybody I interviewed for my book and in previous research projects, who has had a spiritual awakening, loses their fear of death. Not only because they sense intuitively that death is not the end, but also because they can see that their own ego, their own 'I', is not significant in terms of the Universe as a whole. They feel a sense of expansiveness in that they feel connected to something bigger than themselves. They sometimes speak in terms of a feeling of oneness, that everything is one, everything is interconnected and they're part of this connection. They lose the sense of separation from the world."

Those interviewed by Steve Taylor report that these feelings of connection, awareness and expanded consciousness are intense at the beginning and then stabilize after a few weeks at a lower level of intensity that becomes normal, but the transition is a permanent shift. He says, "That feeling of connection, wellbeing and appreciation never leaves and the feeling of being aware of the preciousness of life and the beauty of the world never leaves."

I can see how these expansive states are powerful motivators for the spiritually curious, but those that Taylor has interviewed in his latest book have reached this state of higher consciousness having had a spontaneous spiritual awakening, often as the result of turmoil in their lives, but always unbidden.

I ask about the triggers for these spontaneous awakenings. He explains, "It's usually a sudden and dramatic shift that people go through perhaps in the midst of intense suffering, such as after a bereavement or after a cancer diagnosis. It can also happen after a long period of addiction or incarceration – I found quite a few cases in prisoners – and in soldiers due to the intense stress of facing death on the battlefield. There are also cases where people voluntarily put themselves through stress, like when they do extreme sports where you could encounter death, but in almost every case, spiritual awakening happens involuntarily."

One of the explanations that Taylor offers as to why these awakenings occur to some people but not others in similar circumstances is that, without realizing it, they are ready in some way to be a new self. He says, "It's unconscious, and it's waiting for the opportunity to arise. When the ego dies, that new self just arises naturally, as if it's been waiting to be born, waiting for the space to emerge into. And when the old ego dies, suddenly there is this whole lot of space for it to emerge into."

Dialogues with the Divine

Author Neale Donald Walsch was at rock bottom after a serious injury from a car accident left him unable to work, just as he was going through a divorce. He ended up being homeless and living on the street at the age of 52. He says, "I felt I was in no-man's land, that I couldn't depend on anything that I once thought I knew about life and who I am and why I'm here and all of that." He was, in fact, in a liminal state. It was just as he was starting to get back on his feet – with a low-paid job and a rented room – when he had an unusual spiritual awakening that led to his bestselling series of books.

In the early hours of the morning one day, in a fit of frustration and desperation at the confusing nature of his life, Walsch sat down and impulsively started writing an angry outpouring. "I remember the first question was, 'What the hell does it take to make life work?' I don't even think at that moment I knew who I was writing the question to. It was just a rhetorical question addressed to no-one in particular. And then I began writing other questions. Obviously, there was something that I didn't understand, the understanding of which would change everything. I remember thinking, 'I promise I'll play, just give me the rulebook.'"

It is well-documented that, to his utter surprise, he started to receive responses to his questions, which continued for many months, and these transcriptions eventually became *Conversations with God.* "I realized that I was receiving answers from someplace outside of myself," he says, "because the replies bore no resemblance whatsoever to anything I had heard, embraced or been taught before. Statements were coming out of left field, so to speak, and I had no idea where they were coming from. But I felt this must be coming from God because who else would say such things?

"I realized that the answers that I was being given were healing every false thought I ever had about life, about myself, about divinity and the whole experience. So, I continued with what I understood then to be a dialogue, a conversation with God."

As with any spiritual communication, be it a vision, an answer to a prayer or a clairvoyant message, the big question for me, and for many others no doubt, is always: 'How do you know it wasn't just all in your own mind?' I put this to Walsch, and clearly this thought had also occurred to him. He says, "I can tell you that by the time Book Three began moving through me, I was trepidatious, to put it mildly. I kept asking myself, 'Could I be just making this stuff up? Are these just my ideas arising out of my subconscious?' I didn't want to be misleading myself or anyone else once the first book became massively popular in spiritual circles. I began feeling a heavy sense of responsibility. I deeply scrutinized every word that came off that pen to be as sure as I could be that I wasn't contriving or making it up, even inadvertently. What helped me was an awareness that what was coming through were ideas I'd never had before. Statements that had never occurred to me, much less did I assume that they were on the surface true. The quality of the material, the nature of what was coming through was so different from what I had been raised in or understood in my culture, that I thought, 'Okay, I'm just going to go with the flow and it will be what it is.' I promised that as long as I continued receiving these inspiring messages, I would place them before the public. So, I feel that I kept my promise."

There are now nine books in the *Conversations with God* series and Walsch is adamant that, with *The God Solution*, he has written his last book. Like the people interviewed by Taylor who had spiritual awakenings, the experience he had over 30 years ago has stayed with him ever since and changed the way he lives his life. What put everything in context for Walsch was the answer to his early question, "What does it take for life to work?" He quotes, "The voice said to me, 'Neil, it's so simple. You think your life is about you, and your life has nothing to do with you. It's about everyone whose life you touch and the way in which you touch it. That's how life can work; when you change your mind about what you think life is about.' And that was the most important single message out of 4,000 pages of dialogue that I ever received. And I've tried with a great deal of commitment to live my life that way from that day forward. Ever since, every decision I make, every word I speak, every action I do, every bit of energy that I project is about everyone whose life I touch. When I'm clear about that, my life does work. In the broadest sense life is about me, given that there's only one of us, seeming to have different identities. All things are one. There is only one thing, and all things are part of the one thing there is. So, when I grasped the concept of unity and my unity with every person and every thing, I would actually go into the forest and hug the trees because I got that I am one with everything. From that day forward, everything I did, said or thought came from that place. And remarkable things arose from my sending that energy into the Universe."

Can it be Explained?

For non-believers and those who are cynical about spirituality, the eternal question that is so hard to answer is 'Why would a benign god or higher power allow the atrocities and terrible events that happen on this Earth?' It is hard for anyone to counter this argument satisfactorily, but Walsch has a possible answer: "Yes, we have a dilemma on the planet. If there really is a God, if there is a supreme being, a higher power, then why is the world in such a mess? Who would believe in a power that doesn't do anything to make things better for us? I wrote my final book, *The God Solution*, as an answer to that question. I simply wrote what I understood to be true because it was made very clear to me in the *Conversations with God* dialogues. God's job is not to fix things. God's function is not to do everything for us, but to provide us with the power to do everything for ourselves, to make the choices and decisions we wish to make. That is, God has given us one gift, the gift of gifts, the unspeakable gift – free will – do as you wish, do as you choose. The worst understanding of humanity is the idea that we're separate from God, separate from life and nature, separate from everything, which is what produces the alienation."

As we've seen, science is starting to address the conundrum of consciousness, but when it comes to spiritual beliefs and divinity, there are few tangibles for scientists to work with. Dr Mike Dow told me about research at the beginning of the millennium that identified a 'God spot' in the brain; those who have this are more likely to believe in a God or spirituality. However, that research was superseded by a 2012 study that showed that although there is a neural basis for spiritual experiences, it's not isolated to one specific area of the brain: it is functional rather than anatomical. A sense of the otherworld and self-transcendence is the definition of spirituality and/ or religious sensibility used by the researchers. It is the opposite of being self-focussed and this perception can be generated by additional experiences, including brain trauma, drug states and epileptic seizures.

If science can't provide as yet a solid answer to where higher wisdom might come from, the obvious other place to look was theology. Could the theologians answer these perennial questions? I turned to mystical theology teacher and bestselling author Caroline Myss, who says, "Through the centuries the ways people worship – the gods we pray to, and how we conceptualize God – have changed. Our experience of God is evolving past the half-man, half-god myths of the Abrahamic traditions. The power of the divine is, and always has been, pure power, transcendent of human imagery. But it's only since the middle of the last century that we humans have begun to see past those old images in any significant way. The result is that we are living in a transition, releasing the mythologies of the past and evolving into a new myth, one capable of relating to the psyches and souls of a changing global community."

Neale Donald Walsch believes, "All the world's religions contain great wisdom. My position is that they're simply incomplete. They don't have all the information. We only know a smidgen of what there is to know. I could be wrong about all this, but I think we simply misdefined God. We need to redefine who and what God is and we can do that in two words: Pure Love. God is Pure Love. Of course, I'm always challenged by someone saying, 'We know that God is love. The world's religions agree that God is love.' But God is *pure* love – there's a difference. Pure love requires nothing, asks nothing, expects nothing and certainly demands nothing."

David Olliff takes a similar stance: "If we overwork that sense of what are we and what is the divine, it usually constructs bad theology. If we start with Genesis, we're talking about 'we are made in the divine image', so it must be something we are, something relatable. If we talk of God incarnate, in any kind of way, such as in the Lord's Prayer or the Hermetic tradition, both of which use the simple phrase, 'as above, so below,' there would have to be a very close relationship between human nature and divine nature. If we overplay the otherness, we construct something that leads us to the sort of spirituality that says, 'we need to tread very difficult paths to get to God, to experience the divine and to be within that space.' But these are just constructions. If we think of God as simple, limitless love, then that must be inherently within us. I suspect that, as limitless love, we could not say that the divine is difficult to access.

"So why do we find it so difficult? We find it difficult because we're very good at constructing these ego-based borders, and they are the borders we make ourselves. It cannot be the infinite divine love that is the problem here. The infinite divine love, by its very definition, would have to be very, very easy to access, because it would not be infinite love if it were difficult to access. We think we have to have some Gnostic truth to somehow come to it. The reason it feels that way, though, is we've been very good at building our own ego constructions. Yet the more time we spend in the liminal space, the more time we can allow those borders to break down. That infinite divine love is always present to us. I just don't think we are always present to it."

Accessing the Spiritual Realms

Traditionally, spiritual seekers from around the world have used various methods including meditation, prayer, solitude for contemplation and introspection, and being in nature to commune with the divine, with the gods, angels or with higher powers, depending on their beliefs.

In her latest book *Intimate Conversations with the Divine: Prayer, Guidance and Grace* Caroline Myss offers a very intimate insight into her own prayer practice and urges us all to regain our fluency in the language of prayer in order to renew our connection to the sacred. She says, "Prayer is essential, it is food for the soul, and it is the one required practice of the mystical life. We've removed holy language from our common parlance and the act of prayer from our daily lives. Prayer has assisted humans in the navigation of life for millennia because a direct connection to the divine is essential in navigating life's challenges. Yet how many of us call upon that connection in our everyday lives? Too few of us understand how this connection – or lack thereof – influences our thinking, decision-making and even our health. Too few of us understand that without the grace that is carried by sacred language, our souls will literally starve.

"Prayer is how we communicate with the cosmos; it is the means through which we make ourselves known and heard in the vastness of space. And it's how we receive guidance in return. Prayer is our channel of communication, the direct line between the soul and the divine. We are built for this divine intimacy – and for the awe, belief and inspiration it creates."

Whether you chant mantras, whisper prayers, use prayer beads, have silent conversations with the divine, meditate or even spend time in relation with nature, you are somehow co-creating your reality and conversing with the sacred. As David Olliff puts it, "It is time spent on the threshold of things, the shoreline of things, the border of things, time spent in the liminal. We're afraid of being in the liminal space, because it's difficult to trust enough to give ourselves up to it. Yet the ultimate goal is the surrender of self. 'Give and you will receive' is the ultimate teaching: the more you give, the more you will receive; the more you surrender yourself, the more you will create yourself."

Perhaps it's because we live in a science-dominated commodified society where tangibles and proof are king, but for many, it is the uncertainty surrounding the destination or the recipient of their prayers and supplications that causes them to hesitate. Am I heard? Will I receive answers? Who am I talking to? What am I surrendering to? I asked David Olliff about this and he had some interesting thoughts to share. He says, "I wanted to say something about the business of being uncomfortable with not knowing for sure. The thing about knowing is that it is already a claim of certainty. I think if you had any certainty about God or the divine, whatever you were certain about wouldn't be God, because you would have somehow comprehended it, and to comprehend it is to understand its limits, and if you've understood its limits, it wouldn't be God.

"Knowing is to set boundaries around things. Thus, we're in that business of the liminal again. Wanting to know something for sure is to create a liminal boundary and that's why we don't like the things that are outside that boundary. We think of them as interfering with the purity of our notion of knowing something with clarity. Knowledge is a real issue. Whoever it was that constructed the Tree of Life in the Kabbalistic tradition definitely knew that for sure. When you look at the Tree of Life, there are the ten Sephira, which are aspects of God, aspects of the divine. In between the two aspects of Wisdom and Understanding, it looks like there should be another one. When you look at how the tree is structured, there appears to be a gap, but there are definitely only ten Sephira – you can't just make another one up. The one that is suggested, but isn't there, is Dart or knowledge. The idea being that, when it comes to God, knowing is some element that sits between understanding and wisdom, but it can't itself be a path to God. What's being suggested is that the reason we're uncomfortable with knowing is not knowing for sure. Yet, if we switch it a little, you could say the only way to know God is through unknowing."

On the subject of knowing, you might reasonably think that after an experience such as Neale Donald Walsch's and the success of his books, he might feel fairly confident and sure about who he was conversing with. Yet, even for him, there was always an element of uncertainty.

Moreover, he was unsure as to why he was the one to be chosen to receive these transmissions. This eternal 'Why me?' question troubled him. He says, "I felt I had somehow connected with a source of higher wisdom and higher clarity that I called God. I didn't know what else to call it. It felt like divinity. It felt like divine wisdom. Of course, I asked early on, 'Why me? Why have I been chosen?' And the answer I got was, 'No, no, no, don't think that you are the chosen one. Everybody is having a conversation with God all the time. They're simply calling it something else.' So, you may call it an epiphany, a stroke of genius, a sudden insight, women's intuition, whatever name you can come up with so that you would not be thought of as having lost it, so that you wouldn't be criticized or marginalized in some way for receiving these impulses.

"What you're doing is you're contacting an aspect of life that exists at a level of clarity and wisdom that your mind does not hold, because your mind has limited data – the data that it's gathered since you were born. I came to understand that we are really three-part beings: I am a soul, a spiritual entity, having a body and having a mind, but that this is not who I am. And my soul has all the wisdom of the Universe, because it is not limited to the amount of data that the mind has collected since we were physicalized. The soul is the repository of all the information that ever existed, exists now and ever will exist; the soul is an eternal individuation of divinity."

Liminal Life Lessons

Spirituality is available to us all if we are prepared to step into the liminal territories afforded us by prayer, meditation and other contemplative practices. Here's some of the guidance offered by our experts to help you get in touch with your own form of spirituality.

Expert Inspiration #One

Steve Taylor focuses on the need for a simple lifestyle and a supportive network of people. He says, "In my research, spontaneous spiritual awakenings happened to people who would have classed themselves as non-religious or non-spiritual. In our materialist, secular culture, we don't really understand spiritual awakening. We think of any abnormal states of consciousness as aberrational, psychotic even, so that's why so many people who go through the experience think they are going crazy or they sometimes go to see a psychiatrist who might think they've undergone some kind of psychotic episode. When it happens to spiritually minded people, they can make sense of it much more easily. They have a framework to understand it. It's easier for them and they have a much smoother transition. It's really useful to have that framework of understanding, so if you follow a gradual path of spiritual awakening, it's like slowly walking on a path through a landscape, an ever more expansive landscape and you have time to adjust to it and get used to the climate, to feel at ease in it. If you have a sudden awakening, it's like suddenly being parachuted into this landscape out of nowhere and you think, 'Where am I? What am I doing here?' It's quite confusing and disorientating. Just to have a map, to have a kind of conceptual understanding, is very important.

"The support of others is also helpful. If you're surrounded by a network of supportive people who can give you understanding and support, that's really useful. If they are in the spiritual tradition, that's good. You may have a spiritual guru or spiritual practitioners who can guide you through the process.

"I would also suggest lots of solitude and grounding activities such as spending time in nature, and even in terms of diet, eating a simple basic diet. Living quietly and simply can be really helpful, because sudden spiritual awakening can be a disturbing process, which will settle down naturally in the end. It will return to balance, but you have to encourage the balancing process."

Expert Inspiration #Two

During his dialogues with the divine, Neale Donald Walsch was told the following advice. He says, "I was given an invitation, ultimately, an invitation in three parts. Part one, change the world's mind about God; Part two, give people back to themselves; Part three, awaken the species. It's been made very clear to me that those invitations are not just for me, but for all people who have a genuine yearning to step into the experience and expression of their true identity and their true purpose.

"I always start my lectures with a single question: 'Is it possible, just possible, that there's something we don't fully understand here about God, about life and about ourselves – the understanding of which would change everything?' Then I tell them what I think we don't understand. I'm very clear to tell them at the end of my talk that I could be wrong about it all and not to take my word for it, and I suggest, 'If it serves you, try it. Try living this way and see what it feels like to step into some of these larger understandings that I have.' The largest understanding of them all is that God is Pure Love."

Most importantly, Walsch is keen that people seek the answers to the bigger questions for themselves. He says, "I was told by God in my conversations dialogue, 'Neale, the answer to the question is in the question itself.' So, I have been going around the world for the past 25 years, asking questions and inviting others to ask questions."

Expert Inspiration #Three

Caroline Myss' guidance is that each of us should try to bring the sacred into our lives using sacred language and prayer but she also encourages us to consider that, "Everything, and everyone, in your life is a vital part of your spiritual path. You, in turn, are a part of theirs. This realization may inspire you to live more consciously, more ethically, more generously – or not. But one thing is for certain: your biology responds to the spiritual truth that is active in your soul."

Expert Inspiration #Four

Meditation is favoured by David Olliff as a way to get in touch with your spiritual side. He says, "One of the things that the Eastern Orthodox Church has always been very good at in terms of exercises of the liminal, is the use of icons as a window to heaven. It's quite a nice idea to take an icon and do some meditative work with it – simply staring at an icon for a period of time. Perhaps an icon or an image of the liminal space of the window is a good one, because you get that real feeling of the threshold. Or you could do the same with a major arcana card from a tarot deck. Just meditate on that."

Finally, he would encourage us all to see the mystical and the miraculous in our everyday lives, saying: "The whole creative world is a miracle that we're part of. What I really want of miracles is to be constantly reminded that they're happening all the time. And if I pray for miracles, I'm really praying that I see them, as I sometimes don't see them."

My Chapter Take-aways

- When you search for the spiritual or the divine you are effectively entering into liminal territory. There is no proof or certainty to be had, as non-believers and scientists will point out. For me, the not knowing for sure is challenging, but a kind of intuitive trust is enough to keep me engaged with spiritual practice. My daily practices are loose and fluid, and I like to mix it up. I meditate, but not daily, sometimes preferring to lose myself in mindful contemplation in nature. I pray daily, but in truth I have been known to nod off before I can finish my prayer. I use oracle cards and tarot decks, both of which I feel reinforce my connection with the spiritual world, and I have an altar in my home. I like to honour the moon and the nature spirits, and I love visiting sacred sites, preferably on foot. As you can see, I have a patchwork of practices that bolster my communion with the sacred. Do I follow any formalized religions or practices? No. Can I swear to you that the guidance I receive is from the divine? No. Does placing myself in this liminal landscape of believing without proof benefit me? I believe so, yes.

- Expecting to hear a booming voice from above that tells you in your own language the answer to your prayers may be a tall order. I suggest that when you start communing with the sacred, you manage your expectations and look for more subtle signs of an answer. Many in the mind, body, spirit world believe in common signs of response such as white feathers appearing in front of you, repeating numbers such as 11:11 or 22:22 on the clock, odd coincidences and literal signs jumping out at you pointing to the answers. Just be open to the idea that a response or direction may be shown to you in unconventional ways. The only thing you will know for sure is that you cannot be sure it really is a sign – you just have to trust your intuition and discernment. Choosing a spiritual pathway places you firmly in the liminal ground of being between shores without definitive answers, which is why we can find it uncomfortable.
- Sacred language and practices such as prayer or meditation can help to open us up to spirituality. If sacred language feels strange in your mouth/inside

your head, and you feel foolish searching for
unfamiliar vocabulary, take inspiration from others.
I can highly recommend *Intimate Conversations
with the Divine* by Caroline Myss, in which she
shares the words of her own personal prayers and
guidance. You could attend a spiritual group or join
an online community to get an insight into how you
might like to commune with divine consciousness.
Contemporary prayer is simply a dialogue with
whatever higher power you believe in and an
opportunity for grace and higher consciousness
to enter your world – whatever language/wording
you choose will be absolutely fine if your desire for
dialogue is genuine.

6

TUNING IN TO NATURAL PHASES AND CYCLES

My odyssey of exploration into liminality has taken me through the life changes and transitions that we inevitably face in a normal lifetime to the ultimate transition from life to death, which naturally led me to an investigation into consciousness itself; and from there into the liminality of spirituality and prayer.

I feel drawn to expand my search outwards, from our own internal worlds to the natural world and the cycles of her seasons – those liminal times in our calendar when the natural world is in flux, on the cusp of a new period and all that it might bring.

In the traditional calendar of our ancestors, the changing of the seasons had life-affecting implications and, to mark the importance of these times, the solstices and the equinoxes, fixed power dates in the calendar, were marked with festivals. Solstice literally means 'standstill' – a kind of totality moment – with the summer solstice (21 June) being the longest day of the year and winter solstice (21 December) the shortest in the Northern Hemisphere. Meanwhile, the vernal equinox (21 March) and the autumnal equinox (22 September) are the fixed dates when day and night are of equal length and the sun is directly over the Equator. These dates also mark the start of the seasons in the modern astronomical calendar.

In between those dates fall the Celtic cross-quarter days of Imbolc (c. 2 February), Beltane (c. 1 May), Lammas (1 August – aka Lughnasadh) and Samhain (31 October), and these too were celebrated with fire festivals as times of energetic shift, a moment when change can happen. For the ancient Celts, they signalled the *beginning* (not middle) of a season, with the major two divisions being winter (Samhain), starting the dark half of the year, and summer (Beltane), starting the light half of the year. They are the in-between places, chosen at that time of movement.

Despite ourselves, today the shifts in nature's rhythms, whether that's seasonal, lunar or the cusp times of the day even, are still felt by our inner being. We respond to our environment in an instinctually felt way. Of course, that's not always conscious, but it's still there. The seasons affect our moods and our behaviours. Who doesn't feel more energized in spring and more introspective when the shorter days draw in?

What interests me is that, in the past, people needed an intimate knowledge of the changing weather, seasons, tides and lunar cycles in order to survive. Now, in current times, where our safety and security no longer depend upon knowledge and experience of nature, how and why should we interact with the liminality of these cosmic phases and the cycles of the natural world?

My first port of call was an expert we met earlier. Not only is Alison Davies a professional storyteller, she is also an authority on and writer of folklore and nature, and author of the book, *The Mystical Year: Folklore, Magic and Nature*. I asked her whether the natural calendar and the transitions between seasons still hold any relevance in our modern lives. She tells me, "We may not rely on the different seasons when it comes to growing crops and surviving a harsh winter in the same way, but the transitions still affect us, and how we think and feel, even to the point of experiencing subtle changes in the way we behave and perceive the world. Every cycle in nature has an effect on us because we co-exist. We could not survive without the Sun, the Moon and the stars, without the trees and plants. We are intrinsically linked, so even the subtlest changes within our environment have an effect on us.

"Each season has a very different energy that we can tap into. In fact, we tend to do this naturally to some degree. For example, the summer is perceived as a brighter time, which naturally affects our mood. As a result, we do more, we plan more, we make the most of the days and so we automatically associate the summer with joy, exuberance and activity. Our energy matches the season we are in. With this in mind, it's important to embrace this energy and actively work with it in your life, so that you make the most of the seasonal changes. When you work in conjunction with the natural cycles, you are in the 'flow' and harnessing the energy of the earth.

"The cusps of the calendar year between the seasons represent the crossover, the in-between state, when we move from one type of energy to another. In this state, almost anything is possible. The cycle of the seasons is influenced by the Earth's position in relation to the Sun, and it is this heavenly powerhouse that prompts these changes. The solstices occur when the Earth's axis is closest or furthest away from the Sun, and without the Sun's energy and influence we would not exist. At the solstices of the calendar year, the Sun's influence is at its most powerful and we can sense it all around us."

Since interviewing Glennie Kindred back in 2013, I have been a huge admirer of this highly respected teacher and much-loved expert on natural lore and Earth traditions. She is the author of twelve books on Earth wisdom, native plants and trees, and celebrating the Earth's cycles, including *Earth Wisdom* and *Letting in the Wild Edges*. It felt only natural to talk to her about the subject of liminality in relation to nature's cycles and seasons. Last time I interviewed her, we were in her cosy home in the Peak District and I was fascinated by her garden overflowing with medicinal herbs and flowers. This time, thanks to the pandemic, we had to settle for a Zoom meeting in late autumn – "The perfect time to let everything settle back down into Earth," as she describes it.

Observing the seasonal and natural cycles may no longer be essential to our daily lifestyles, but she is adamant that they still have a huge role to play in our lives. She says, "The survival thing is not so important in terms of physical survival, but I think in terms of our mental, emotional and energetic survival, it has never been more important. Our survival is on the line, and I believe it's because we've become disconnected from nature. So, it's very much about survival, and how we reset our initial condition to become a new, reconnected type of human being again, because the disconnection has played havoc with us. Those liminal times, dawn and dusk and those other liminal times when we just have a moment and we feel totally connected, are so important to us. They remind us of who we are, as part of the Earth. It's part of the rewilding of the human, isn't it? We're in this process at the moment of rewilding ourselves, re-finding our connection to nature and our unity and interconnectedness, rather than the separation that we've been conditioned to believe. There's a lot of the liminal within that context."

Certainly, when I was still editing *Kindred Spirit* magazine, it was evident to me that the rewilding movement was gaining momentum. People are now more open to having a deeper and more instinctual way of being within themselves and the natural world. I welcome the proliferation of interest and courses if it helps to reconnect people to nature and their ancestral heritage. You can now attend nature workshops ranging from gardening for biodiversity and planting native hedgerows and woodlands, to creating wildflower areas and wildlife ponds. Most heart-warming to me are the workshops that encourage us to reconnect with our wild man and wild woman archetypes – the part of ourselves that is a rebellious seeker of inner truths, drawn to spending time in nature and being more connected to our surroundings.

Glennie Kindred tells me that she has always focussed on the cusps of the year, known as the cross-quarter days, and the powerful lessons they hold for us still. She explains, "The cross-quarter festivals of Imbolc (February), Beltane (May), Lammas (August) and Samhain (end of October/November) are the seasonal peaks, and then the year tips over into a new season. It's those liminal points really between when everything is full, but everything is also on the move.

"The community used to come together and light fires on the hilltops at cross-quarter and lunar festivals. The equinoxes are balance points. They're points when day and night are equal and there's a stillness and a balance in that. Whereas the solstices, where you're at the extreme of the cycles, and the cross-quarters, that's when people came together because it's the fullness that is about to change.

"I use the festivals to reset myself and to bring myself back into my spiritual alignment. I set my intention to that very thing and I take that opportunity to realign. I've been doing that now for 30 years. Every six weeks, at the festivals, I take a day out, at least a day, sometimes two days. That's for my reconnection to the Earth and reconnection to my spiritual path, and it's a fantastic practice. You could say that I had this great good fortune to be able to devote my time and energy and thinking to these things, but I've made it so, in a way, by setting that as my intention."

Tuning In to Natural Cycles

Personally, I can vouch for feeling the changes of the seasons. Summer is definitely a time when I need less sleep; I can still be found sitting in my garden by the chiminea late into the night and I am happy to rise earlier to start my day; whereas in winter, I could happily be in bed with my book at 9pm. I imagine I am not alone in being attuned to these liminal times of the year. But I wondered what subtle effects we undergo at other less familiar cusp times such as the cross-quarter festivals, for example, and would I even notice? How do we tune into these calendar phases?

Danu Forest is the author of several books including *The Magical Year: Seasonal celebrations to honor nature's ever-turning wheel*. She describes herself as a traditional wise woman, a seer, a druid witch and priestess, and an Earth-based Celtic shaman. Suffice to say, she has dived deep into the theories and practices that work closely with the powers of the land. She was also a regular contributor to *Kindred Spirit* magazine. I felt sure she would be able to add to and shed light on the relevance and effects of natural cycles on our daily lives. "The cusps are some of the best times to tune in to the natural rhythm. What I've noticed with my students, and my own personal life, is that at that time, it's more of an 'allowing' rather than a hard and fast effort – allowing that awareness to unfold in yourself and taking that time to pause and just notice the in-between time, notice the shift, as that's when change can really come and when you can steer change. Whether that's how you are going to navigate your day or how you are going to make life choices; it's feeling that in-between place and shifting it from there.

"The in-between times have always been associated with spirit time. The Welsh call them *Ysbrydnos* – spirit nights. You know, those liminal times of the day and of the year are always times when we pick up on wider things, whatever they may be and however we interpret them: earth energies, ghosts, fairies or nature spirits. In medieval times, they were described as the 'doorway' times of the year – and I like that. It's about a liminal process, perhaps when we can become aware of the wider nature of our reality, as opposed to those normal times when we are just getting on with the practicalities of life."

Thinking about it, my grandmother always lit a candle in the window at Halloween (Samhain in the Celtic tradition) to ward off bad spirits. Both her and my mum were psychic, and we would light the candles and focus on them to encourage stillness and connection, and to honour the ancestors. She said this was the time when the veil between the worlds is at its thinnest and when connection to the spirit world is at its easiest. So, Halloween being a cusp time – that now makes more sense to me.

Yet, we don't have to wait every six weeks to connect to the liminal times in the seasonal calendar. According to Forest, we can practice on a daily basis at dawn and dusk if we choose. Forest describes it, "There's that feeling when the light changes at dawn and dusk. I mean, in reality, most of us are much more familiar with dusk, aren't we really? We all love the idea of dawn, but how many dawns do we see compared to dusks? At dusk, there's that feeling of the day falling away behind you, and a still point coming, an awareness coming, a space coming after the day. As we enter into evening, we've got that sense of more of an internal spaciousness than we would have had during all the activity of the day."

Getting into Nature at Liminal Times

I am a great fan of walking. I think of it almost as a physical meditation and I can lose myself in contemplation roaming on the moors above our home with our dog for hours. Weirdly, my favourite time of the day to walk is at dusk. Coincidence or instinctively feeling drawn to the possibilities of this liminal time? I'm not sure.

Glennie Kindred is also a big fan of walking but she favours striding out on her own as she finds a dog's energy quite disruptive. What we both agree on is that we love to be on our own in nature. She says, "It's a fantastic feeling to go for a walk on your own, but especially at dawn and dusk. It's powerful. It's connecting. It makes you feel alive.

These are the liminal times of the day. So, they're when the night is at its fullness but about to spill over into the day; and the day is at its fullest but it's about to spill into the night. They're exactly the same point. I couldn't explain why they're so powerful, we just have to stand in awe and wonder. Walking alone and absorbing and observing nature. It's as simple as that really. Then the change comes over you.

"For me, at that point, I feel that I'm connecting to my wise inner knowing, my instinctive self, my intuitive self. It's part of me that, if I don't give it space, I can't hear. We've all got it. Our intuition is always rising to the surface, but we often don't notice it, or dismiss it as not being important or as true as our logical, rational mind." Walking or just being in nature, especially at the liminal times of the day or the seasons, is the perfect time to connect and listen to your own inner wisdom, then.

Setting Intention and Creating Ritual

Throughout history, people have celebrated key dates on the seasonal calendar, usually linked to farming traditions and to the pre-Christian religions. Take, for example, Harvest Festival, which was customarily celebrated when the harvest had been safely collected in, which coincidentally also happened to be the Sunday nearest the harvest moon. This is the full moon that occurs closest to the autumn equinox. In the calendar of the ancient Celts, the first day of summer, or Beltane as it was called, was celebrated with bonfires to welcome the new season, and in many rural settings, on this day, they still dance around the maypole and crown the May Queen. These folklore festivals continue in a watered-down version all over the world, so I wondered how important it is to use ritual to connect at these liminal points in the calendar?

In Danu Forest's view, traditional rituals and ceremonies are wonderful, but not essential. She believes we can make use of our own little rituals. In her case, one of her favourite rituals started when her son was young. "When he was a baby, I would spend every dusk with a cup of tea outside in my back garden. Just one cup of tea, watching the bats fly around and taking just ten minutes. It was sacred to my day. My husband had the baby and I would just breathe and reconnect. It can be just as powerful in those still times.

"I've got a long-term student. He's an old guy who lives in Wales. He's a native Welsh speaker. To be honest, he doesn't really go in for ritual and magic and that sort of thing. What he likes to do is every day, he sits by his fire and he smokes a pipe and he talks to the gods. He talks to the Welsh gods, Gwyn ap Nudd especially, who is part of the mythologies of the mountains around where he lives. He sits there and he chats, as one old guy to another. The insights that come from that sacred checking-in space are immense. They are probably some of the most powerful things I've ever heard, purely from allowing it to happen, from giving the opportunity and allowing the relationship.

"The rituals are lovely, but that reaching out for a relationship is the key thing. There are definitely additional things to be gained from adding on the structures of ritual, but at the very least, the core of it has to be the relationship. It has to be feeling that shift and reaching out – now is the time. There's such riches and such power to be found in these really simple acts at these liminal moments. Just that pause, that reaching out to spirit or to your own inner voice."

To Glennie Kindred the actions themselves are not what makes a ritual powerful so much as the setting of an intention. She explains, "When you set your intention, you are already in a sacred space. I formally create sacred space at each of the eight festivals, connecting to each of the elements, speaking aloud my connection to those elements outside of myself, and how that resonates for me as part of that element. The power builds up when you do that, and you create a sacred space. You can do many things in sacred space. You can leave sacred space open all day and go for a walk. It alters you. You reset yourself so that you're in a more receptive place. By creating sacred space, you shift your perception.

"At dawn and dusk and the seasonal cusps, your perception is shifted by what's happening around you; you can feel it. I think it's something to do with us recognizing that we're more than this logical surface reality; that we have these feelings and we connect through our heart and our sense of wonder and awe. It shifts us. Unfortunately, a lot of people don't give themselves the chance to experience these shifts."

The Roman Empire officially adopted Christianity in 380 BCE and, from there, it spread north and west into Europe. In 386 BCE a law was passed declaring that those 'who contend about religion ... shall pay with their lives and blood.' For the previous 70,000 years, people's principal belief system was Animism, believing that spirit lived in everything from trees and streams to animals and nymphs. The early Christians believed that the pagan beliefs were infected by demons and were sacrilegious, and the might of the Roman Empire was used to purge paganism – a trend that continued into the mid-19th century. While the vast majority of ancient literature that espoused the views of the pre-Christian doctrines was destroyed, and many artefacts too, paganism managed to maintain a foothold among the common people. It seems that the wise women, faery doctors, cunning men or shamans of the village would use whatever physical locations were to hand to connect to the landscape and to find their source of power. At times of trouble, they would connect to the spirits by leaving out offerings for the faeries perhaps or asking for guidance on healing the sick, and they would seek out liminal places to practice. Forest confirms that this is what she has found in her own research into Celtic and Druidic practices, saying, "I hadn't realized how prevalent it was for shamans, wise women, etc to go to the crossroads, in Wales and in England especially. Practitioners would go and work in the cross spaces. They might cast a circle, or they might not, but essentially, they would go out at night and they would go to the crossroads to practice whatever it was they were doing. It's spelling it out on the land – you're at a crossroads, and it's physically represented. It's that inside and outside connecting somehow. And again, that liminal space in the landscape; it could be the edge of the lake, the edge of the sea, a mountain or a cave but if you didn't live in a dramatic landscape, it was the local crossroads. It's a hub place, where it's not quite this, not quite that, but lots of possibilities can come from it."

Lunar Transitions

There is one more natural cycle that may well have an influence on our bodies and minds that I would like to explore and that is the movement of the celestial bodies, the stars and the planets, but principally it is the moon phases that draw my attention. Like many other women, in particular, I feel a definite connection with and attraction to the Moon, and I have an app on my phone that tells me about which phase of the Moon we are experiencing. But that doesn't explain how the different liminal phases of the Moon affect all of us here on Earth.

Almost as soon as the questions popped into my head, I thought of contacting moon-kissed astrologer Yasmin Boland who is author of the book *Moonology: Working with the magic of lunar cycles*. Boland, who has taught thousands of women how to work with the Moon's endless beautiful cycles, principally using new moon wishes and full moon surrender ceremonies, tells me, "By being aware of the lunar cycle, we connect with the planet, we go outside, we get some fresh air, we get some moonlight. You know, moonlight is really important for people to bathe in. We bathe in moonlight in my household as often as we can, because it's the play of the light of the Sun on the Moon, and the sun is the very yang, masculine energy and the moon is a very yin feminine energy. So when you get moonlight, you're actually getting a combination of the yin and the yang, and it's very balancing. It's good for you.

"Being aware of the moon cycles is really about honouring the planet and being in touch with that side of ourselves, which can otherwise get lost in our hermetically sealed, air-conditioned or centrally heated boxes with our electric lights and our microwave ovens and our computers. It's a way of reconnecting, and when we reconnect, we start to reconnect with our basic powers – the powers that we were born with. You get back in touch with some kind of primordial power that everybody has, but especially women, and it comes from the Moon. There is such a thing as moon power."

Much of Boland's moonology teaching is based on her research into both Celtic and Hindu wisdom; to this day many people in modern India still let astrological movements influence their daily lives. Yogi and mystic Sadhguru, who is founder of the Isha Foundation, says, "In India, every day is counted and how the different positions of the Moon can be used for human wellbeing is an established part of the culture. To do anything, it would be useful to be aware of where the Moon is because it creates different types of qualities and energies in the system. If you bring a certain level of awareness and perception, you will see the body behaves slightly differently for every moon phase. It is very much there in both the male and the female body, but it is more manifest in the female body. The timing with which the Moon goes around the planet and the cycles that human beings go through within themselves, are very deeply connected." Given that the movements of the Moon can cause whole oceans to rise, and that we are made up of 60% water, I can see how physically the Moon's phases and gravitational pull might have an impact on us. But emotionally? How does that work?

He says, "The Moon pushes your energy in a certain way. If your quality is joy, you will become more joyful on full moon days. If your quality is love, you will become more loving, if you are meditative, you will become more meditative. If you have a mental illness, that can also get enhanced. Whatever your quality is, it gets enhanced because of the full moon.

"In the mystical world, human perception and the Moon are directly connected. Adiyogi, the first yogi, wears a crescent moon upon his head like a jewel. This is to indicate that he is at the highest level of neurological stimulus. The neurological development is the most significant aspect of who we are. And how stimulated, active and balanced our neurological system is, is directly related to the phase of the Moon."

Glennie Kindred admits that the moon phases affect the timings of her seasonal festival ceremonies. "The quarter festivals, that is the solstices and the equinoxes, are astronomically fixed dates, but the seasonal cross-quarters aren't at all. I've always said, it's got nothing to do with the calendar date. I think it's got more to do with the Moon. Some of them lend themselves better to a full moon energy and some lend themselves better to a new moon energy," she explains.

Of the use of rituals, Boland says, "When I first started working with the Moon, I started doing new moon intentions and full moon forgiveness and I'd write out my lists. But quite a few people wrote to me asking if there were any rituals to go with this. So, I came up with my own ideas for the new moon intention setting but, for the full moon work, I looked closely at what they do at the ashram I visit in India. They do big fire ceremonies, what they call *yagams*, so I started to do my version of those. For a long time, I didn't feel I could do rituals; I felt I wasn't qualified. My teacher in India also gave me an idea for a ritual, which was to get petals from flowers and to chant. I think just doing that and realizing how powerful that felt, and how much that impacted other people who enjoyed it gave me confidence. The thing with rituals is that we don't do rituals for the divine, we do them for ourselves. The divine doesn't need our rituals. The rituals are here to help us connect and to step into the liminal."

I'm completely on board with the rituals. Who doesn't feel moved by sacred ceremonies? But, why not do them whenever the mood takes you? Why wait for specific times? Boland shares her view on how the tipping points in the lunar cycle can influence us, and why we should celebrate then. She says, "In a funny way, the lunar cycle is a constant stream of liminality. The Moon is in a constant state of flux. And its changes from one phase to the other are a very slow thing. With astrology and moonology, these things don't switch on and off like light switches. We give them names – the new moon, the full moon and the quarter moons, but it's really just a continuous, endless cycle. They're actually the result of the play of the shadows of the Sun on the Moon. Back in the day, at a solar eclipse, when everything went dark, people would think the sky was falling in and think it was a very bad omen. We now have the benefit of knowing that eclipses happen for various astronomical reasons, and they're nothing to be scared of. They are, in a way, portals and opportunities, which open up for people to step through.

"One of the biggest benefits of tuning in to those different phases is the fact that it actually puts us back in touch with the planetary, the lunar and the universal cycles. Depending on where we live, it's not always very easy to spend time, especially at night, getting in touch with the cycles. You know, for most people, the seasons come and go and we don't pay much attention. The change of the seasons has always worked off the ingress of the sun into the four cardinal signs of Aries,

Cancer, Libra and Capricorn. So when the sun moves into the sign of Aries, in the Northern Hemisphere at least, it's spring; when the sun moves into Cancer, it's summer; when it moves into Libra, it's autumn; and when it moves into Capricorn, it's winter. In Australia, where I grew up, the legislature decided that was all far too complicated. Rather than having it based on that, which is around the 20th of the relevant months, they now say summer doesn't start around 20 December, it starts on 1 December. It's another way to disconnect us from the seasons and from the natural cycles."

Seeking Reconnection

Since all those I've spoken with are convinced of the boost to our wellbeing that tuning into the liminal opportunities of the various phases of the seasons and the planets can offer, and if these ancient wisdoms and practices have such proven benefits, I couldn't help but wonder why we find ourselves in such a disconnect and why these practices have virtually died out? I raised this with three of the experts that I interviewed. Their responses were unequivocal and uniform: the rise of the patriarchy was largely responsible.

Although Yasmin Boland is clear that we are better off in so many ways in our modern world with the technological, scientific and medical advances that have made our lives easier and saved us from terminal diseases, she wants us to be more in touch with the feminine and to bring the knowledge back. She says, "Remember, all this knowledge about the Moon was stamped out 500 years ago because they kept burning the women who made their tinctures and potions by the phases of the Moon at the stake, or drowning them or hanging them. No one knows how many women were killed but obviously the practices stopped. But now it's coming back. Somehow, there is some connection with women and the Moon and power.

"There's something mystical and mysterious and women are doing it again. I started doing moonology 25 years ago now, and I was honestly a lone voice in the wilderness. Now every woman is out there under the new moon, making wishes and setting intentions and doing release work at the full moons. Women are realizing that this stuff works. It doesn't matter how many times the patriarchy might try to make fun of us; this stuff works. That's probably why it got banned the last time."

Kindred says, "When people have those sorts of powerful moments at those liminal times, perhaps at a waterfall or with a tree, and they feel that shift in perception in themselves, it can be very frightening. It's like, 'Whoa, my reality has wobbled. I'm not prepared for this.' And it's true, we haven't been prepared for it. In fact, we have got a long history of such things being ridiculed. We've all got this very bad conditioning that makes us frightened of it. It doesn't encourage us to be open to it in a state of benevolence."

There are several reasons, according to Danu Forest, as to why we have become disconnected from our natural abilities and why we're so uncomfortable in these liminal spaces. She says, "Perhaps because we are so reliant on certainties with our scientific, materialist thinking, we rely on just one way of looking at the world, and we find security in that. Once you're living your life on rails, the idea that actually life has got more possibilities, that can be very frightening if it hasn't been opened up to you from an early age. You see it with a lot of women, in particular, who get to a certain age, perhaps menopause or their children are grown, and suddenly, they've been on these rails their whole life, they've been sitting with certainties, and then one day, it cracks open for them. It can be difficult – they will change, and it could be an amazing opportunity for them. They know they are going to be their authentic selves now, finally. Generationally, we are taught to do what's expected. We find security in what's expected and don't really see ourselves in relation to those liminal places in ourselves. For centuries, we've been taught to fear them. But when you see the penny drop with these women after they have had those initial experiences and they realize that they've experienced something that women have been experiencing on these lands for an impossible amount of time to calculate, that expands their entire sense of self and life."

The final word goes to Yasmin Boland, who says of our desire to link to the phases and cycles of the seasons and planets, "People crave that moment of devotion or that moment of ritual. In terms of liminality, we are multi-dimensional beings; we're not humans on the planet disconnected from everything. I believe we are all connected to all life everywhere. That eventually means we're connected to what you might call our higher self, or god/goddess, the great spirit – whatever you want to call it. In terms of liminality, it's about being somewhere in between this 3D person that we grow up thinking we are and this higher consciousness, which we are connected to. Maybe we are somewhere between the two when we are doing the ceremonies.

"I do think that this transition women have made from being burned at the stake to now coming out and standing up again, it's a very liminal thing that we're in right now. Who knows where we are along the timeline, but we've been a long time in the liminal."

Liminal Life Lessons

Without really understanding it, many of us feel the subtle influences of the changing seasons and the planetary cycles on our minds, bodies and emotions, especially those of the Moon. If we actively choose to tune in to those phases and make use of them to navigate our way through modern life, or to connect more to our inner guidance, rather than repress or ignore them, it seems to me that we can maximize the potential of these liminal times in our day and our calendar and incorporate the possibilities that lie within these liminal times into our own lives.

Expert Inspiration #One

Glennie Kindred is convinced that, "We can't just carry on using our minds to work everything out. We've got to actually feel it. Experiencing it makes it real. It's all about our relationship with the Earth and with ourselves. It's all in the flow. There's nothing to beat getting out there and experiencing that relationship."

In order to feel again, her recommendation for all of us is to get into nature: "Even if you're in a town, you can step out into the park, you can sit with your back against a tree, and just find that stillness in yourself, not chatting (well, you can hear your inner chatter), and then sinking into the earth to try and let that inner chatter settle and to find a sense of stillness. Because, when we fill our outer world, which we have big time, there's no room for the inner world to rise. We have to make space in the outer chatter in order to hear inner wisdom and our inner voice. There's nothing finer than sitting with a tree, wherever that tree is. It's all very simple. There's nothing complicated about any of it.

"It's also about setting the intention to take a day out, if you can, to mark the festivals and check in with yourself. If not, then a half day or a couple of hours, whatever it is.

"I've also been keeping a moon diary for the last 18 months. I just write, like automatic writing, not really thinking about it, just letting out whatever comes at the full moons and the new moons – that's every two weeks. It's made me more aware of the moons, especially the full moon, and I find myself looking for it, where it is in the sky in relation to my house, and going out into the garden. Moonlight is absolutely amazing."

Expert Inspiration #Two

In order to be more in tune with natural cycles, Alison Davies says, "I'm a great believer in moving with the seasons and taking inspiration from the natural world. I think it's important to acknowledge what each season means to you personally and how it makes you feel. We are more connected to the natural world and the transition of the seasons than we might imagine, but it takes a moment of stillness for us to realize this. At the changing of the season, I suggest taking time out to simply stop, breathe and take in the changes around you.

"Performing rituals to acknowledge the changing of the seasons is a way to connect with the energy of the natural world. I actively look for nature's blessings every day: small things, like a beautiful sunset, the heat of the midday sun on my face or the rustle and crunch of autumn leaves underfoot. If we're open and engaged with our surroundings, then we'll automatically tune in to those natural cycles."

Expert Inspiration #Three

Danu Forest would encourage each of us to try and balance our outer lives with our inner life. She counsels, "If you can listen, if you can heed your inner voice, take some time every day, become aware of greater possibilities, the rich aspects of life, be with yourself quietly, then you have the ability to navigate yourself. It's a lifelong challenge in its own right. It's an ongoing challenge in relation to what's going on around you. But having that ability, having that inner skill, makes so many more things possible."

Expert Inspiration #Four

Yasmin Boland tells me that she may be considered a tough teacher, but that there is no excuse for not getting out into nature. She says, "Unless you're living somewhere that's war torn where you literally can't go out the door because there are bullets firing, there's always going to be some nature somewhere not too far away. There's always going to be a park, you know. I live in West London, and our local cemetery is actually quite a nice park; we go there a lot. I will definitely hug a tree. We also live near the river, so we go down to the river. There's always somewhere to be in touch with the Earth. You can always do that.

"I do have people who say to me when I'm talking about doing a full moon forgiveness list and burning it, 'Well I live in an apartment, and I can't really do a fire like you do in your backyard. Can I just use a ceramic pot and put my paper in there?' and the answer is, 'Of course you can.' Don't be limited by these things. These things are trifling. There really is no excuse to say 'I've got no nature.' Just being under the sky is being in nature.

"When I do my full moon ceremonies, I always get out. Often, the skies are overcast in the UK, and you can't see the full moon, but if you can't see it on full moon night, you can see it the night before or the night after. Even if the skies are overcast, you still get the benefits and you're still bathing in the moonlight. But, as with everything, intention is important and assists. It's always good if you have the intention of 'I'm going to go out there. I'm going to get some moonlight. I'm going to put on some beautiful music. I'm going to do a meditation and just soak up the moonbeams because I want to get more balanced.' The intention really helps."

My Chapter Take-aways

- Journaling is a great way to reflect on the natural cycles – ask yourself simple questions and then write down your first intuitive response as a good starting point. At solstices and equinoxes, consider how you are feeling and note down your responses. Get used to tuning in to subtle changes in your body and emotions, then you can expand your journaling to include other cusp dates in the seasonal calendar.

- Why not get yourself a lunar chart for your wall or make a note of the Celtic festivals and try to become familiar with these dates in your calendar? Celebrate them in whichever way feels right to you.

- Ritual can enhance the spiritual experience, but setting an intention and just sitting with stillness and nature at these liminal times is enough to feel the benefits. I like to walk barefoot in my garden on dewy mornings and warm evenings to help me ground myself. I also have a little ritual of heading outside and thanking the full moon for her blessings on full moon nights while trying to let go of what no longer serves me. At the new moon, I will sometimes light a candle on my altar and set my intentions for the coming month. Nothing grand – just changes or things that I would like to see in my life.

- Much of the traditional wisdom, especially of the wise women, in relation to natural and lunar cycles is making a comeback. Perhaps one of the workshops or courses in rewilding might be right up your street?
- I only have to look at the sacred geometry of fractals, patterns and shapes that nature repeats all around us in flowers, trees and plants to be in awe.

7

WILDERNESS, THIN PLACES AND PILGRIMAGE

I now have a better understanding of the effects that natural and universal cycles can have on us and the liminal opportunities they can offer. This leads on to one of my all-time favourite topics, and probably the inspiration for this book: liminal spaces or, as they are perhaps better known, the thin places in the world.

It's thought the ancient Celts and early Christians first coined the phrase a 'thin place' to describe those rare locales where the veil between this world and the other world is thin. It's somewhere that transcends the senses and where the distance between heaven and Earth is shortest.

For me, it was feeling drawn to certain spots where I felt a mystical, ephemeral and mysterious atmosphere that is almost palpable that first got me interested in the liminal – places where, for a few blissful moments, I can feel the spine-shiver of something beyond myself that is also beyond words. I've felt it on the edge of a glacier in Patagonia, on a solo hike in the Scottish Highlands, but also at the Nubian pyramids in Sudan, the deserted palace in Fatehpur Sikri in India, and St Martin-in-the-Fields church in London. So, although I am usually stirred by this sense of otherworldliness that defies description when in remote and rugged landscapes, I can also experience it in certain man-made places.

A thin place is anywhere where you lose your bearings, where thoughts fall away and a numinous quality remains; it feels special and ineffable. Thin places are often sacred spaces – the Blue Mosque in Istanbul, the standing stones at Avebury Henge, St Peter's Basilica in the Vatican City, Lindisfarne Priory on Holy Island or the Golden Temple in Amritsar – but they need not be. A thin place can be anywhere that moves you into the liminal, where you feel captivated, disoriented, charged, as if anything were possible, connected to an indefinable power that is larger than you can perceive.

What unites all these experiences, irrespective of locale, is the reaction in me that they engender. Wild moor or hallowed ruin, I feel moved, engulfed almost by a sense of the mystical, of greater possibility, of the eternal. I get goosebumps just thinking about it. Even once I have reluctantly left (it's hard to draw away from these places), an odd somewhat spacey feeling remains for quite some time. It's not a high – it's more of a calm centredness that is addictive.

As a result of this mysterious and nebulous quality, some people do not feel comfortable in thin places. Others, like me, are drawn to them. Glennie Kindred feels the same way. She says, "I look for thin places. I love them and I know quite a few. I actively court them, because they make me feel more alive, more than I was before I stepped into them. I feel excited by them. I get that other people perhaps feel fearful, but I'm not particularly fearful in my nature. I'm very open to receive. I learned years ago, with shamanic journeying and things, that you enter with benevolence and you receive benevolence. Whatever we give to the moment, we receive back from the moment. I enter thin places with love in my heart and the fear is not there. And if I do ever sense fear, then I get out, because then that's instinct. So, it's knowing yourself really."

I asked her what she thought a thin place might be, even knowing that it is an almost unanswerable question. Nonetheless, Kindred has a go at putting her feelings into words. She says, "I use the expression, 'more than'. It's a place of increase, a place where there's connection to more than what I think I am. They're places of expansion really, but it's inner expansion. It's not outer expansion. You couldn't put your finger on anything in the outer. You can't rationalize it. It's an inner threshold where we connect to being 'more than'. It's not a very good way of explaining it, but it makes sense to me because I become more than this outer shell of the person that I am in the outer world. It's a place to find that balance between the inner and the outer, that's one of the keys. I'm courting this liminal world. Not many people are actually courting it. But if they did court it a little more, there's a wealth to be found."

A world-acclaimed expert in Feng Shui and space clearing, Denise Linn elaborates on the power of place for me. She says, "Not all places on the land are the same. There are some places that just naturally – perhaps because of the formation of the mountains and the rivers or if you know the form system of Feng Shui – are more advantageous than other places. A lot of places where they talk about vortexes or portals, these are places where someone planted intention. Something powerful happened, maybe a powerful ceremony was held, and there is a residual energy that continues to be renewed as more people are drawn to it. According to the hills and the land, Mecca wouldn't seem like a natural vortex, but it is definitely a vortex now because of the millions of people that have sent energy to that place, and the intentionality and ceremony and focus again and again. There are some places that will energize you and some places that will deplete you. The sacred sites tend to be the places that energize you. In those places, mystical things can occur. In those places, there's a thinning of the veil between this realm and the next."

Phyllis Curott writes and lectures on the embodied spiritual wisdom of Mother Earth. I have always been a huge fan of Curott and her work, and was delighted when our paths eventually crossed. As an attorney, one of America's first public witches, and founder of the Temple of Ara, America's first and oldest shamanic Wiccan tradition, I felt sure she would have knowledge about thin places and our relationship to them. In a lengthy and fascinating discussion, she says, "There are places that are particularly potent in the energy of the Earth, and they've always been so. You can sense it. Whether it's a well or my garden, everywhere has a spirit of place, but in some places, it's particularly potent, and we should pay careful attention.

"The first time I went to Australia on a book tour, I knew I had to go to Uluru to make an offering. When we landed, it was raining. It never rains. We got in the car and the guy drove us up there and then started to drive around. To his surprise, I asked him to stop at this one spot. I walked in and it was green, with water sneaking down the rock into this area that was growing. I took a little water and blessed myself and made my offering. Long afterwards, I found out that it was this incredibly sacred site that is supposedly where the rainbow serpent comes down. How did I know that? My heart knew that, and the part of me that welcomes life as the chance to be in liminal space to do that. I went to make an offering and the space welcomed me. There are mysteries; may our hearts be open to them, and open to what they have to teach us.

"The witch persecutions of the 1700s and 1800s severed people from their relationships with medicinal plants and psychotropics and the use of drumming for altered states of consciousness, but it also severed their relationship with holy places, places on the Earth that hold powerful energy, but they're still available to us. There are energies that flow around the globe that connect us all."

Explaining the Energy of Thin Places

Scientists have sought to explain thin places by suggesting that electromagnetic fields, generated by certain kinds of rock, could make a location feel odd. Some talk about an 'emotional residue' of certain places – so, a location where a disaster took place would have a sad vibe perhaps. All potentially possible, I suppose, but it doesn't go anywhere near explaining the special experience I've had when I've encountered a thin place.

The nearest thing to an explanation for me is the definition of a ley line or energy line, as first discovered by amateur archaeologist Alfred Watkins in 1921. These power lines often coincide with the timeless routes used by our ancestors over thousands of years. The places where ley lines intercept, the thin places, were special to our forebears and they often sited monuments and stone circles at those spots. As Denise Linn says, "There's a deep current of energy that illuminates these places, and a pilgrimage to any one of them can connect you to the sacred space within you."

Author Victoria Preston, who wrote *We Are Pilgrims: Journeys in Search of Ourselves*, says of pilgrimage sites, "The thing that I've looked at over and over again, and never really resolved, is why we have such a powerful sense of place? Why a place takes on this greater significance? You could say some of these pilgrim sites are very ancient, like Rome or Jerusalem or Mecca, but why? In Yorkshire, they talk about sheep being 'hefted' to the land. So, it's very difficult to get certain sheep to move down off the hillside because they are hefted to that spot. I think human beings can be hefted to a place. What we've done with this phenomenon of the magnetic pull of a place is the same as we do with everything that humanity touches – we elaborate it until it becomes highly ritualized, highly ornamented, yet more and more significant. We take some fundamental emotion, like a desire to stay in a place, and we create around it, we build around it."

Travelling the Sacred Routes

Travelling migratory routes probably started in prehistoric times, and following routes to sacred sites was certainly a well-established practice by the time of the Celts, and later, by the early Christians. By then, such journeys were known as a 'pilgrimage'.

Although we are familiar with the role of pilgrimage in a religious context, pilgrimage has served to connect and reconnect people and places from prehistoric times to the present. Research at a site near Stonehenge in England suggests that Neolithic people travelled and drove animals hundreds of miles to the site to be slaughtered for ritual feasts and to attend cultural and sacred events. Yet that doesn't explain why pilgrimage is still relevant in a largely secular 21st century. I wondered if Preston could shed any light on why we remain drawn to travelling along ancient sacred routes. She says, "We still have some animal impulses. As Chaucer said, 'When spring comes, when April showers do prick the drought of March, then we long to go on pilgrimage.'

I think there's something very instinctive about it. It's so engrained in society and actually, setting aside the Neolithic and the trans-migratory practices that were the original fundamental driver of pilgrimage, all the major religions have pilgrim festivals orientated around the tipping points of the year, like the point between winter and spring or the point between the end of summer, autumn and the beginning of winter. These are the liminal moments in the calendar, and actually, we rejoice in those moments in the modern world too. In those moments of deep uncertainty, those liminal moments, we have a festival, we take a pilgrimage, we take time out for reflection."

When Denise Linn was explaining about a vision quest, she pointed out to me that it can take the form of a retreat in nature, or it can be a pilgrimage. She says, "Although a pilgrimage has a different form than a traditional vision quest, often the outcome is the same. On a static vision quest, you seek answers to soul-searching questions through an inward journey, whereas on a pilgrimage, you discover your life's meaning through the outer journey. You can think of a pilgrimage as a mobile vision quest, and you can call for a vision on your pilgrimage. Visions and insights can be received in the same way as on a stationary quest, but the idea of movement while on the quest, and being able to watch the signs and observe what happens along the journey, to me is very powerful. A pilgrimage is a physical journey through time and space, but it also stands as a powerful rite of passage that can touch you very deeply."

Motives for Undertaking a Pilgrimage

I was curious to find out what distinguishes a pilgrimage from any other kind of journey, so I asked Victoria Preston for her view. She says, "There are different stages of pilgrimage. Stage one is the impulse to go. Stage two is setting out along the road and being in that liminal space, which I always think of as a kind of apex – you're not on this side of the mountain and you're not on that side of the mountain, you're just walking along a ridge of nowhere-ness. I'm sure lots of hillwalkers have the same feeling, which is the liberation that comes from being in the natural world on a journey, on a walk, and feeling that you're moving through time and landscape and space. Then stage three: the moment of arrival. A lot of pilgrimage writing is really about the destination. You know – this shrine, this crypt, these artefacts or these rituals that happen in that place. And that's not to dismiss them. For example, it's very moving to read the accounts of people's experience of the Hajj (pilgrimage to Mecca) when they feel themselves to be part of a much bigger humanity, and any sense of us being divided and different falls away. The idea of being part of a much bigger whole is very profound. The final part of pilgrimage is what happens when you return home and how your journey then informs the way you proceed in your own day-to-day life."

It strikes me, having digested Preston's words, that the sacredness of pilgrimage sites is an important inducement for many pilgrims, but almost as important are the lessons that are learned in that transitional space of the journey itself, after you have left home but you haven't yet arrived at your destination. The pure essence of pilgrimage is that what is revealed on the voyage is as important as what awaits you at the end of the journey.

I am still unclear though, in my own mind, about what drives modern non-religious people to undertake a pilgrimage. I can see why religious devotees would travel to sites that are sacred to their specific religion, and spiritual seekers might wish to visit their own places of spiritual significance, but why do secular pilgrims set out?

David Olliff believes, "I've always thought of pilgrimage as an interior journey. *The Wizard of Oz* is the analogy. Dorothy goes out in search of a way home, only to find she could get home anytime she wanted. The lion is in search of bravery, only to be given a medal because he is already brave. We go out in search of thin places because we discover ourselves at the thresholds, where the water meets the land, for example the edges of lakes and rivers. These are the borderlands, and the wilderness is a borderland. In the borderlands, we meet the other and we meet the other self – they are places of encounter."

One school of thought that Victoria Preston related to me is that there are only two motivators for people to go on pilgrimage – either to say please or to say thank you, that is, to ask for something or to give thanks for having received it. So, does she buy in to this theory that motivation for pilgrimage is gratitude at one level and fear at another level? She says, "It's much more to do with liberation. What you're looking at is this escape from the everyday into this sort of liminal space. I think that is much more what we are doing now with pilgrimage, particularly secular pilgrimage. It's really about liberation, the quest for enlightenment, the quest for some kind of exceptional insight that we cannot get sitting in our living rooms."

So how would Glennie Kindred define what constitutes a pilgrimage? She says, "When you're out on the land, if you go out with the right intention, that's pilgrimage. One of my favourite things is to step out with a sense of pilgrimage for a walk. It may only be an hour's walk, but you walk as a pilgrim – connected."

Preston agrees, "It is precisely the intent that makes it a pilgrimage. Whether your intention is to come closer to your god or closer to yourself, or to be liberated from yourself, the intent is absolutely critical. For me, it is the defining thing. Actually, our intentions, in a way, are informed by our own spiritual parameters. If you are a practising Christian, your intent for your pilgrimage, even if it's the salving of grief, is framed by your Christianity. For novelist Jack Kerouac, who wanted to get away because his work was not being published, his intention is framed by his practice of Taoism, for example. So, he chose to go up onto the mountain, which is a Taoist practice, rising up to get as close to the heavens as possible. So, I think intention is nine tenths of the law."

I wondered if a pilgrimage has to be hard. After all, there always appears to be an element of self-challenge so as to show true devotion, and the most devout religious pilgrims walk barefoot or travel parts of the route on their knees. The most famous pilgrimages – El Camino de Santiago, the Abraham Path, the Hajj, The Pilgrim's Way, Mecca, the Nakahechi Route in Japan or St Olav's Way in Norway, to name but a few – are all considerable distances taking several days or weeks. Does Preston think pilgrims must challenge themselves? "Does it have to be hard? No, it's what is in the mind while you're on the journey that is important," she concludes.

Denise Linn believes, "Discoveries don't have to come through struggle. Sometimes it's a gentle recognition." Phyllis Curott adds her voice to the conversation. She believes that you have "to go into nature with a measure of openness, willingness, interest and gratitude." She then tells me how, at the age of 50, she took a pilgrimage with a friend as guide to a thin place – a canyon in the Lower 48 states – in the middle of winter. "My request in being there in this wild place was to be in liminal space; to let go of the past, and to be fully present and to feel the presence of the Great Mother, Mother Earth, and to undergo some healing because my marriage had recently ended. And to see my way forward to the next work that I would do."

When she came out, she was blessed with her next agent and her next book deal. She says, "I came out of the canyon and everything was waiting for me."

As Victoria Preston says, "What was interesting to me was how similar pilgrimage is across all faiths; there are more similarities than differences. Not just across faith, but across time as well. This sort of connection to the natural world, this feeling of being part of something bigger in the universe, the Great; whether you describe it as your God or not, it's an acknowledgement of being part of a big unknown force that guides the Universe. When you're out in nature, you feel that whether you're Christian, Jewish, Muslim or whatever."

Qualities of a Pilgrim

All the experts seem to agree that one of the greatest positives to come out of being in thin places, at sacred sites or on pilgrimage, is the sense of connection it gives us, either with nature or with our higher selves. The other thing on which there is total agreement is that intention is crucial. However, I wondered whether other qualities are required in order to experience the full benefits of being in these places and/or en route through or to them as a pilgrim?

Peace-pilgrim, lifelong eco-activist, author and former editor of *Resurgence & Ecologist* magazine, Satish Kumar, now 85 years old, is well-known for undertaking a peace pilgrimage from India to Moscow, London, Paris and America in his twenties. Walking with no money and depending on the kindness and hospitality of strangers, Kumar delivered a humble packet of 'peace tea' to the leaders of the four capitals of the nuclear world. He clearly understands the importance of intent, but what other qualities are required of a pilgrim, I asked him?

"I would say that all of us need to live on this Earth as pilgrims and not as tourists. For the tourist, the mindset is to take, not to give. Tourists give money, but that's nothing. Even as they take, they are never content. Tourists live with expectations and expectations are never fulfilled. Whereas pilgrims do not expect anything. They drop all expectations and all anxieties and fears, and they accept life as it comes. Whatever is given to them, it's a gift. And they accept with gratitude. So, they drop expectations and celebrate acceptance. And when you accept life as it is, then pilgrims walk and participate. When you participate in life, you radiate your love, you radiate your compassion, you radiate your joy as a pilgrim. We should live humbly, more like pilgrims, and celebrate the bounties and the generosity and abundance of nature. On a pilgrimage, you are active and yet you are contented. That active contentment is the quality of a pilgrim.

"Being a pilgrim is an important attitude of life. When you are a pilgrim, you take time off and go out walking in nature. Everything is holy. Land is sacred. Trees are sacred. Mountains and rivers are sacred. Animals too. So, when you go on pilgrimage through mountains, forests, along rivers, through hills, you are in sacred space. And then you are one with the Universe. There is no separation between you and nature, between you and the Universe, between you and the Earth," says Kumar.

I asked Phyllis Curott how we can tune in to the sacredness that Kumar describes and that is so often to be found in thin places and on pilgrimage? How do we return to right relationship? She says, "When we go with humility, even when asking for something, but offering our appreciation, our respect, our humbleness then nature responds to us, because it's alive and it has a consciousness – it has energy, it has wisdom, it embodies the divine. When you bring your attention and you breathe in a very simple way, which is part of the way I practise and teach now, you're engaged in communion with creation and the experience is numinous. You could say you're entering liminal space. If liminal is what's unknown, that would be nature, wouldn't it? We don't know it at all. It is profoundly liminal. We have to open ourselves; we have to acknowledge that we don't know. We have to invite something greater than our own capacities to work with us. But, if we're willing to enter the natural world with an open heart, a sense of gratitude, with an acknowledgement of how small we are, and believe you me – go to a canyon and you know – then nature is constantly giving us everything that we need to rediscover how to live in right relationship. We have to learn to pay attention. The things we can do are quietening the mind, opening the heart, being sincere in inviting the wisdom and the blessing and the energy of nature and of the sacred to enter us and make its magic."

Rituals, Practices and the Weight of Expectation

If you follow this advice and plan to spend more time in nature in the hope of finding a thin place, or to arrange a pilgrimage of your own, I suspect, as a novice, you are most likely to visit celebrated sacred locales or to tread trusted historical pilgrimage routes. Yet, I feel there is an inherent danger in this plan; is what one person finds a thin place the same for everyone? Or is thinness like beauty – very much in the eye of the beholder? Eric Weiner in his spirituality travelogue, *Man Seeks God,* would suggest so: "You don't plan a trip to a thin place; you stumble upon one. But there are steps you can take to increase the odds of an encounter with thinness. For starters, have no expectations. Nothing gets in the way of a genuine experience more than expectations, which explains why so many 'spiritual journeys' disappoint."

This ties in with Satish Kumar's view that to travel as a pilgrim rather than as a tourist, you should set out with intention and without expectations, but it doesn't help in deciding where you go. A top tip from Mindie Burgoyne's website, thinplacestour.com, may prove useful in this regard. She says, "You can look for thin places, but frequently they will find you. Once you set your spirit on finding them – they will actually find you. There is an intrinsic, mystical spirit woven into the fabric of nature, landscape and sky that calls out to every human heart – if only the heart is willing to listen."

I suggest that friends with whom you feel a kindred spirit may well be able to recommend a place or a route, or you may just find yourself drawn to a name that inexplicably captures your heart and imagination. That's a good place to start, since some of the known sacred places have such a weight of expectation on them that they may disappoint. I'm sad to say that I felt nothing remarkable when I visited Stonehenge, yet the standing stones at Callanish on the Isle of Lewis and Isle of Harris in the Outer Hebrides blew me wide open and left me mesmerized. Try to keep an open mind, is what I'm trying to say.

Victoria Preston says that the same applies to heading out on a pilgrimage. "When I went to Delphi, the site was crawling with tourists. I stayed overnight, while most tourists go back to Athens. I was sitting in a café, saying, 'What's special about Delphi? I'm not feeling it.' Someone said I should go early the next morning before the tourists arrived. The following morning, I went very early down to the Temple of Athena Pronaia, which is further down the slope of Mount Parnassus, and it's much older than Delphi. Then I was like, 'Now I get it. Now I can feel it.' Of course, I had really psychologically prepped myself and it was dawn. As we know, dawn is one of those liminal moments where you're very open to different experiences."

So, does the weight of expectation lie within us rather than having anything to do with the power of the place, I ask her? "We all travel with our own baggage, right? We take that luggage with us wherever we travel. Alain de Botton touches on this in his book *The Art of Travel*. To paraphrase, he says that the problem with going on holiday is that you go on holiday with yourself. Whatever you have in terms of luggage, it comes with you. In a way, when we go on pilgrimage, we are trying to shake off all that baggage. We do it both literally and metaphorically. For me, one of the great things of walking through Italy was just having a backpack with one change of clothes, a pair of binoculars, water bottle and sleeping bag. You're completely self-sufficient.

"In a way, we are looking for something. We want something to happen. You're in this liminal space and you're open. You've cast aside all worldly considerations and you want to feel something. So, you've got your emotional eyes peeled as it were. You've got heightened awareness. Whatever it is that's within you, you are open to connection."

Sacred spots and thin places hold power that affects each of us to a greater or lesser extent, but undoubtedly, our preconceptions of these places can amplify their effects. This was certainly the case for traveller and broadcaster Ben Fogle when he visited the windswept Inner Hebridean island of Iona for the first time, during his latest travel documentary series, *Scotland's Sacred Islands*. Iona has been a sacred place since St Columba arrived on its white sandy beaches with 12 followers in 563 BCE, built his first Celtic church and established a monastic community. Once settled, the Irish monk set about converting most of pagan Scotland and Northern England to the Christian faith. When Fogle visited the island, he found himself in tears. He admits that this may in part be due to nominative determinism, since he named his daughter after the island, and says, "I wanted it to be a beautiful, profound place, and I found it very moving – not necessarily in an absolute religious context. I found the whole experience very comforting."

It seems we can invest all sorts of special power and meaning in pilgrimage and place, and often we reinforce this with ritual. I asked Preston if the ritual of a journey or practices at a sacred spot can add to its significance. She says, "You can't pull ritual apart from pilgrimage. Human beings are very ritualistic animals. For example, we do the anticlockwise circling when we go on pilgrimage. People on Hajj do it – anticlockwise, seven rounds in the direction of the sun. People on Croagh Patrick do it – seven times sunwise around the cairn on the hilltop. When we do these rituals, we believe it's an act of superstition. It has value to us. Rituals are a way of taking ourselves into the zone we want to be in mentally. In a way, ritual is what we use to translocate from the mundane into the exceptional."

Phyllis Curott discovered core shamanism and Wicca in her twenties, and recognized that both disciplines retrieve and recreate the practices of our Euro-indigenous ancestors. She says, "What I learned quite quickly is that good practice is practise that works! These techniques are universal. They're shared. They may have different cultural nuance and form, but they've been shared by indigenous peoples all over the world for thousands of years – people who have maintained right relationship with the planet, who experience it as their mother, as a spiritual teacher, who know that it's numinous and liminal, alive and entirely holy and sacred. Casting of a circle is the creation of a liminal space. When you enter it, you're entering the womb of the divine feminine, and your mind and heart are open, the magic flows into you. The goddess appears, if you like. All indigenous people work in circles. They honour the four directions, and the Sun above them and the Earth beneath their feet. They recognize that we humans have this remarkable capacity to be aware that spirit and worlds are one, and that part of our purpose is to help maintain the balance between spirit and world."

Feeling the Benefit

Personally, I feel drawn to pilgrimage and to thin places because of the charged effect they have on my spirit, but I decided to ask each of the experts what they believe can be gained from being in the wilderness, at thin places or on pilgrimage.

Phyllis Curott starts the discussion by talking about the power and gifts of being in nature generally. She says, "I spend as much time as I can in the natural world, and I pay attention. I pay attention to the seasonal changes because within them is a deep spiritual wisdom about the cycles of life, and about how we're meant to live. Being in nature makes us better, makes human nature better. It simply does. From a scientific and psychological perspective, we know that when you spend time in nature, your cortisol levels drop, your heart rate drops, your stress diminishes. As important, if not more important, is that when that happens, your sense of awe floods you. Simply being in nature inspires awe and makes us more altruistic. Human nature is better in nature. I have endless stories of the magic of being in the natural world, of the numinous just abundantly expressing itself again and again."

The benefits of pilgrimage are many and manifest, according to Kumar, but the most important is that of the potential for fulfilment of your true potential. He says, "When you are a pilgrim, and when you walk like a pilgrim, and when you put your love into it, that's when you open to self-realization. It's through love that you receive self-realization. You are a love being, a spiritual being. So, self-realization is to let go of your judgemental ego and to express your true being to humans and nature equally."

Meanwhile, Glennie Kindred advocates that we each seek out our own thin places to help us to feel something greater than ourselves. She says of the possibilities to be found in liminal space, "Throughout history, this connection to our imaginations, to our inner abilities, our healing abilities, our creativity – all of that is part of being in that liminal place. It offers us an expansion into our inner selves, which are so undermined and undervalued. I feel as if there's so many keys to our humanness to be found there really. To become lost in your inner self is really good. That's why I paint and make things. I can lose hours and I like that. If you are able to find that stillness and kind of empty away, ground, earth yourself, then there's room for the other, if you want it. It feels good and it particularly feels good if that happens when you're out on the land with a tree or with a spring."

I couldn't agree more. I actively seek to be alone in the places that move me as it helps me to commune with nature but also with myself. These opportunities for solitude and self-contemplation, and to feel something bigger than ourselves, are so rare in our busy modern lifestyles, so when I do set aside time for them, they have even more meaning. I cherish the ineffable feeling of awe, wonder and connection that thin places give me. In these places, on these pilgrimage walks, it feels as though I am touching the sacred.

For Denise Linn, she experiences something similar, and says, "For me, personally, and it's probably different for every person, it's almost like a remembering; a remembering what is important in life, a remembering who I am, a remembering why I'm here, that I am a part of something vast and wondrous. I am a new sprout on an old root. That for me is powerful because it's so easy to forget."

Reaching for Connection

I suspect from everything that I've been told that many people, when they set out on pilgrimage, wittingly or otherwise, are seeking some sort of connection, either to nature or to the higher self or to the sacred. There is a yearning to connect to something greater than the mundane. Victoria Preston certainly recognizes the desire for communion with a greater force. She says, "We feel ourselves reaching upwards always. This idea that there's a veil between us and some mysterious defining force I think is true. If you read accounts of astronauts, as I do, because obviously, space is the final frontier of pilgrimage in a way, they look back at Earth and they have a completely different view of existence by being able to step outside it into space. And in some places, and at some moments, we feel ourselves to be living on a planet, whereas in our daily lives, we feel ourselves to be living in a house. It's a different feeling.

"I had this feeling very profoundly in Canada. I looked at the landscape and was totally in awe. The fact that it had been formed by huge powerful forces, and that you realize in that thin place that you are on a planet. In that moment, I thought to myself, 'I wish I believed in God.' It was such a profound feeling that this has been created somehow, that you're almost looking for the signature on the bottom."

I know exactly what Victoria Preston means. There have been occasions when I have felt almost overwhelmed by the majesty and beauty of the natural world. While exploring in Patagonia, we found ourselves kayaking on Lake General Carrera, the vast, turquoise-watered glacial lake that straddles the border of Argentina and Chile. The surrounding mountains were reflected in the calm surface of the lake and, at that moment, I could see the hand of the divine in the creation of our world. I felt the sacredness that pervades that remote spot. Yet, connection does not have to be on such a grand scale. Walking in local woods, I will often pause to connect with the Earth, to touch the trunk of a tree to tune in. Modern life conditions us to be disconnected from nature and the sacredness of the liminal spaces that we find in the natural world, and yet when I take time to reconnect, to heal that separation, I feel so much better in myself.

Phyllis Curott reiterates the importance of healing that separation, saying, "We've forgotten that the natural world is our practical teacher and our spiritual teacher. When we come into the presence of the liminal, it's all about touching the potential that comes from inside of us, but also comes from something greater. When we honour it and respect it, then it starts to trigger us to do that in harmony.

"I've never found anything to be afraid of in the liminal. Witches spend their time like everybody else, you know, but part of what we do is move between realms of spirit and this world, because we know that the two worlds are one. We become skillful at seeing spirit in this world, as well as skilfully entering realms of spirit. It's an extraordinary way to live. It really is. Everybody has the capacity. Some people are better at it than others – witches are more interested, we're more devoted to it and more attentive to it – but everyone has this capacity.

"For all of us now, part of our purpose has to be healing the wound in ourselves, healing the separation from nature, from the sacred, because they are one, and healing the world that has been created out of this separation. Coming back to starting to see the natural world as an embodiment of spirit."

Perhaps we can leave the last word on the indefinable mysterious magnetism of thin places to pilgrim of peace Mahatma Gandhi, who said in his 1931 *My Spiritual Message to the World,* "There is an indefinable, mysterious power that pervades everything. I feel it, though I do not see it. It is this unseen power that makes itself felt and yet defies all proof, because it is so unlike all that I perceive through my senses. It transcends the senses."

Liminal Life Lessons

From time immemorial, people have been drawn to thin places – elemental landscapes or sacred sites where you feel an immediate connection with place and with spirit, where transformation can happen. In setting out, with the right intention, to visit these power sites, we find ourselves as pilgrims, and as many insights can be gained from the liminal journey of a pilgrimage as can be drawn from its sacred destination.

What tools and practices do our experts use to connect to these deeply inspirational, sacred places and journeys?

Expert Inspiration #One

Glennie Kindred, lover of nature and thin places, suggests that you can start off modestly. She says, "It's as simple as stepping out really with awareness and gratitude. It's about the flow of energy. Step into that place where you feel. Gratitude opens the heart; when your heart is open, you are more connected. Creating connection, being open to receive – it all begins with gratitude. Be thankful for the seasons, thankful for nature. The more you're thankful, the more you appreciate, and the more you appreciate, the more you're connected, and the more the separation is healed."

Expert Inspiration #Two

Satish Kumar lives with a pilgrim's attitude to life and asks each of us to do the same. He says, "If we follow our own heart, follow our own spirit and are truthful, compassionate and kind; if we respect nature and live with nature in a contented way, and live with other humans with humility, then we can have a state of mind that is a pilgrim's mind."

Expert Inspiration #Three

Victoria Preston's advice is simple. "In times of deep uncertainty, take time out for reflection." What better way than walking alone into the wild or on a pilgrimage, which is her chosen method.

Expert Inspiration #Four

Denise Linn places her emphasis on the intention behind the time you spend on a vision quest or pilgrimage. She says, "Although the vision quests and vision pilgrimages I led were usually three days, there are many different ways that you can quest. There is value in taking time and being methodical and different realizations will emerge. But if you only have a day or an hour, use that day or hour. Just be present with life. Be mindful in that time, be open and inner results can come. Remember results occur outside of time and space. They can occur as a direct result of your intention.

"If you believe in talking to spirit, you can say, 'Hey spirit, I only have an hour now. I know that's not a lot of time, but I am just asking that you're present, and this is the most glorious, amazing hour of my life.' I mean why not? Why not hold that intent rather than thinking, 'Well, I have only got an hour; not much can happen in an hour." Be focussed with your entire intentionality that this is going to work, and when your heart is open and your intent is clear, results will come no matter where you are or how long you have."

Expert Inspiration #Five

There are lots of simple practices that we can incorporate into our daily lives to help get back in touch with nature, according to Phyllis Curott, who uses the following techniques herself and also teaches them. She says, "Simple practices of working with the elements of nature, learning how to breathe, and being fully present help us to rediscover how to live in right relationship. There are techniques that open perception to shift us from the beta consciousness that we mostly spend our time in, which is that survival mode, to the relaxed alpha mode, such as meditation, which clears and quiets and opens the mind; and shamanic techniques that create the theta trance state, like shamanic drumming, which opens the mind further into the liminal so that you can see the sacred.

"The trick is to develop a simple skill set that can help you, that can enhance your innate capacity to listen, to see. Offerings are very important, actually. Even if you're not mastering practice, the simple going with gratitude into your garden, into the park, into the woods, into a field and making an offering of something that's useful, like water or bird seed or corn, is a way of beginning to establish a healthy relationship with place.

"So, my work for the next part of my life is to get people to breathe properly and drink water in the right way and to lie on the ground. Do these simple things that everybody does, no matter your religion, your politics, your ethnic background, your nation – it doesn't matter."

My Chapter Take-aways

- What sets a pilgrimage apart from a walk/hike is the intention, so it's useful to think about a purpose before heading out as a pilgrim. What question is it that you want answered in your life at the moment? What do you want to attract or let go of? Or do you want to give thanks for something? Once you have set your intention, your journey has a purpose and becomes a pilgrimage. You may not get the answer to your question on the walk or even afterwards, and you may get other unexpected insights, but setting an intention prior to setting off is always a good idea.

- There are great websites, books and articles that list some of the more traditional pilgrimage routes. One of my favourites is the charity British Pilgrimage Trust (britishpilgrimage.org), which shows routes and distances in the UK – a fabulous resource. Yet, you can always choose somewhere less obvious that has meaning for you – a favourite childhood family holiday destination, a loved one's grave. And remember, distance is immaterial on a pilgrimage – it's the intention that counts.

- There are recognized thin places and sacred sites in the world, but given the choice, I like to discover my own in less trodden places. That said, I have a bucket list of well-documented destinations that I'd like to visit, which include Iona Abbey in Scotland, Taktsang (Tiger's Nest) monastery in Bhutan, Koyasan (Mount Koya) in Japan and the Great Mosque of Djenne in Mali. Oh, and I'm keen to strap on my walking boots for a pilgrimage along the Beara Way, County Cork in Ireland.

- Since Pagan times, people have honoured the Spirits or Powers of Place by making offerings. If you feel moved to make an offering in order to establish a positive relationship when at a thin place or sacred site, then make sure it is biodegradable and well thought out. Bird seed is an option or a libation of spring water or vibrational essences is another suggestion.

8

OUR NATURAL WORLD
ON THE BRINK

Our journey together through this enquiry into liminal space and what it means is almost at a close. There is just one last area that I would like to delve into and that is the glaring example of liminality that affects each and every one of us – our very own planet rocking on the brink of ecological disaster.

Our world hovers in the liminal space between timely and sufficient restorative action and decline into irreversible damage from emissions, burning fossil fuels, deforestation, over-farming and use of nitrogen fertilizers. There is a groundswell of public opinion and some NGO and government action toward greener initiatives, but no-one yet knows for sure what the outcome will be. Too little too late or just in the nick of time? I speak with a handful of experts as we sit in the uncomfortable liminal space of not knowing what the future of our planet might look like and if we are yet doing enough to save her.

When I think about this topic, I'm minded of a line from the docudrama, *The Age of Stupid* by Franny Armstrong. That film is set in 2055, when the world has been devastated by rising sea levels and various natural disasters and an archivist is examining videos from 2008 to understand why humans didn't stop climate change before it was too late. At one point, the narrator Pete Postlethwaite says, "Why is it, knowing what we knew then, we didn't act when there was still time?" It seems appropriate that we ask ourselves – and the experts – this question now.

Firstly, I ask if it is too late or if there is still time to turn things around. Documentary filmmaker and activist Bruce Parry says, "I'm hopeful. We're definitely at a crossroads, but I've been saying we're at a crossroads for some time. So quite how big this crossroads is, it's hard to discern. I definitely think it's possible that we can come out the other side, and that what we could come out with could be unbelievably beautiful. I mean like paradisiacal. I just think that we as a species are amazing. I've witnessed how humans can interact with each other in unbelievably good, positive and harmonious ways. That is possible for us, if we choose, but we need to want it and to know about it. I should qualify that by saying I'm not a hopeless romantic. I've seen things happening with indigenous peoples that are destructive to each other and the planet. So, I'm not a romantic just because I've spent time with tribal people. I'm actually very much the realist."

I also ask eco-activist and former editor of *Resurgence & Ecologist* magazine Satish Kumar if he is optimistic that we are acting in time to avoid a disastrous outcome. He had given a speech at the ChangeNOW international summit for change in February 2020, and was invited to speak at COP26 (although he couldn't attend), so I knew he would have strong views. He says, "I am an activist. To be an activist, you have to be an optimist. If you're a pessimist, you can't be an activist. I am always hoping some transformation, some change, something is happening. COP26 is not a destination; it is a milestone on the journey. It is very good that so many people from around the world – politicians, business leaders, NGOs, all the people who have gathered together – are talking about climate change and the importance of nature, that is very good.

"This is a milestone on a long journey of transformation, but when you have a juggernaut like the European economy, American economy or even the world economy – to turn that whole economy around cannot be done overnight. So, it's a good start. What we need now is a strong grassroots people's movement. This is where the pressure will come. In *Resurgence & Ecologist,* we started talking about climate change 30 years ago; I published articles by James Lovelock back then; Schumacher was writing about it 40 years ago; Teddy Goldsmith was writing about it 45 years ago. These pioneers have laid the path. Now governments and businesses are going to put trillions of pounds into renewable energy and into some sort of green economy.

"If you look at the world, the human impact and human footprint is so severe and so heavy that we haven't left any nature intact. We have brought an end to nature. If humanity doesn't turn now at COP26 and after, then we are doomed. Therefore, I have to be an activist. I have to be an optimist. I have to have hope and I have to do something, so that this juggernaut can be turned around and we can change the direction."

Even though COP26 may not have delivered on all its promises, it was still a step forward. Public pressure and awareness continue to grow around the world and it is clear that we are waking up to the fact that something has to be done about the existential threat that the climate crisis poses to humanity. COP26 had been hailed by some as our 'last best chance', and was later condemned by many activists as a failure for not meeting all the goals that the summit had set for itself, but that doesn't mean that we should just give up. We need to keep the pressure on our governments and to continue to do our own small bit to reduce our carbon footprint.

The most uplifting thing for me is that when change happens, it can be very fast as it gathers momentum. We have all seen what would once have been considered inconceivable U-turns by governments on environmental issues. We simply do not know which actions will trigger a breakthrough, so we have to keep fighting and to keep hoping.

Some years ago, attorney and activist Phyllis Curott's prognosis for the planet was less optimistic. In fact that's an understatement, but she explains that her view has changed somewhat over time. Now she tells me, "I don't know if we have crossed beyond the tipping point yet. We may have," she says. "I fell into a deep depression for quite a number of years because I thought that we had crossed over and that there was nothing that could be done. Also, that there was nothing that I could do as an individual. But Mother Earth shared with me that there are ways that it can still work. I realized it was my job to write, and to share the knowledge. So, I'm writing a book and I'm teaching about what we can do as individuals."

Curott shares some of her tips for individuals at the end of this chapter. Bruce Parry adds his qualified agreement, saying, "It's only in the coming together of all of the individuals that we have a movement. It's in the coming together that the hope can be found. On our own, yeah, it does feel difficult and hopeless. That's why things like XR (Extinction Rebellion), for all its faults, and all of these other movements are galvanizing for people.

"For me, it's system change that is the only answer. It has to be absolute, complete and utter change of everything. That might only come from deep shock. We've just had a little shock with COVID, and all our leaders are saying, 'Back to business as usual.' It's madness; business as usual is what's killing us. At the moment, we're going completely in the wrong direction.

"I don't think we are taking it seriously at an institutional level. Left to the institutions, there is no hope. The power structures are so addicted to their own power that they can't let go and this lies at the heart of the problem. The only solution comes from the awareness of the people, of everyone else. And that's difficult because it feels so hopeless and helpless and all the narratives that we are being fed by the media are taking us in the wrong direction, almost 180 degrees in the wrong direction. Every story that we have – more fame will make you happy, more money will make you happy, more goods will make you happy – these are the things just filling the void of loneliness, and filling the void of loss of community and filling all of these voids that make us run around in circles. So, we're all out of kilter.

"In a way, we've been too successful at creating the world that we want, and we're only just waking up to realize that what we want is actually not good for us. We want all these things and they're actually really destructive. Yet it feels terrifying to let go of that and to go in the other direction because that feels like a sacrifice. What I've experienced is that actually we're even happier with the simple things. We don't need a new Lamborghini to feel happy. It's not what people talk about on their deathbeds."

Meanwhile, Satish Kumar is more confident that individuals will make the difference. He says, "The young people's movement has got everybody coming together now. Greta Thunberg is just one of the hundreds of young people in every country who are waking up and raising their voices. In Africa, America, China and Europe, hundreds of boys and girls of school age are demanding change and they're making a big difference.

"There has been a build-up of the environmental movement over the years. Pioneers like Friends of the Earth, Greenpeace, WWF – all these organizations have been building the movement. Extinction Rebellion and other radical organizations are also raising their voices. So, the great river of the ecological/environmental movement is made of many hundreds of small tributaries, and these tributaries are all coming together, and now suddenly it's becoming a big flowing river."

Collective Responsibility

Talk of our collective and individual accountability nudged a memory from an earlier conversation I'd had with Dr Eben Alexander about Near Death Experiences and consciousness. He'd pointed out that if we reject the nihilistic and materialist science thinking and accept that consciousness is more than chemical reactions and electron fluxes in the brain, then that means that we have free will and with that comes responsibility. I asked him to expand upon the implications. He tells me, "To deny a sense of responsibility can be very damaging. Of course, you see that writ large in the current climate emergency. I mean, we've already fallen off the edge of the cliff. We're already in deep trouble. All we can do is respond as quickly and efficiently as possible to get rid of our addiction to fossil fuels, stop polluting, stop putting plastic out there to choke all life to death. We need to be responsible as a species and individually."

Yet, although all the experts I spoke to are rightly and seriously concerned, most feel that there are some glimmers of hope. Dr Alexander says, "I often say that there's a good news/bad news thing with climate change. The bad news is that it's getting worse so much more quickly than anybody ever anticipated. Every annual report is much worse than the one a year earlier. It goes into the unprecedented territory of 'Oh my god, can you believe this is happening?', but that's also the good news. It's gotten to where only the most flaming ignorant idiot will be denying that climate change is destroying our planet and that humans are responsible. That is becoming very clear to all of us."

It occurs to me that one of the pillars of treatment for addiction states that recognizing that you have a problem is the first step in getting help. Drawing a parallel, perhaps that is why only now that we are acknowledging that the world is in this liminal place where the scales of the planet's future are starting to tip, are people beginning to explore inventive and positive solutions to the problem.

Eco Initiatives

The more I started to look into it, the more people and groups I found who have used the creative breathing space of the liminal to come up with some amazing and innovative approaches to solving the climate change challenges we face right now.

Recently, I watched the first televised award ceremony for the Earthshot Prize, launched by Prince William the Duke of Cambridge, in 2021. As well as identifying and rewarding evidence-based solutions to the biggest environmental problems the planet faces over the next decade, "The Prize aims to turn the current pessimism surrounding environmental issues into optimism, by highlighting the ability of human ingenuity to bring about change, and inspiring collective action."

The programme showcased some astonishingly inventive and positively genius ideas and enterprises, and this is just one example among many of the steps toward reversing global warming and redressing the balance with nature.

Sadhguru's Conscious Planet initiative focuses on the ecological problem of soil exhaustion. He says, "Right now, UN statistics say that we may have enough agricultural soil for only 80–100 crops. This means it is a matter of 40 to 50 years. After that, there could be severe food shortages and rich organic land or soil will be the basis of battles and wars on this planet. Unless we start now, we will be heading for a disaster. If we take concrete action in the next five to ten years, then we could turn the soil around in the next 25–30 years. But, if we wait to take action after 50 years, it will take 100–150 years to turn the soil around. That means four to five generations will go through terrible states of life because the soil is in a bad condition. Only in preserving the quality of the soil will the quality of the planet and life endure. This is the greatest legacy we can leave for our children.

"We are living in a time when we have to think of protecting the things that have always nurtured us. This is the first time in the history of humanity that we have to talk about protecting the planet. Never before did anyone have such an insane idea that they had to protect the planet. The planet always took care of us. Preserving and nurturing this planet is no different from aspiring for a good life for ourselves, because there is no good life without a good planet. Right now, we are looking at ecological concerns as some kind of an obligation that we have to fulfil. It is not an obligation. It is our life."

Mending our Relationship with Nature

Many of the global initiatives that came up in my research – such as the Trillion Trees project – which pledges to protect and restore one trillion trees by 2050 for the benefit of people, nature and a stable climate – place heavy emphasis on restoring the balance in nature. With that in mind, I wonder what having time at the crossroads, sitting in the liminal space of change, has shown our experts about the actions needed to preserve the natural world.

When Satish Kumar talks about reverential ecology, an approach he has promoted for many years, he is connecting the spiritual dimension with the ecological dimension. He says, "We start by changing our attitude toward nature. At the moment, we think that nature and humans are separate. Nature's out there – our mountains, rivers, birds, animals and insects – and we humans are separate. We are the rulers of nature; we are the superior; we have colonialism and nature's our colony. We can exploit nature as much as we want – it is only a resource for the economy. Whereas, if you take the Indian culture, where trees, rivers and the Sun are worshipped and nature is considered sacred, we revere nature. Therefore, I want to say that we need to change our attitude toward nature.

"First and foremost, we have to say that nature and humans are one. We are nature. There is no separation. Nature is life itself. Once we have this attitude change, where we see nature as sacred, together with a reverence and respect for nature, then we will not put all this plastic in the oceans, we will not cut down the rainforest, we will not put any animals in factory farms and treat them with cruelty. We will not put chemicals, pesticides and herbicides, or any other poisonous substances into the soil, or carbon dioxide and methane gas into the atmosphere. All that will change only if we change our attitude. Nature is not a means to make money, nature is sacred, nature is our mother and nature is our life. We are not separate from nature. That is the fundamental change we need to see."

Once again, the liminal makes an appearance, as Phyllis Curott, who broadly agrees with Kumar's approach, explains to me that paradoxically, we've swapped 2,000 years of civilization, where the three Abrahamic faiths have told us that God is transcendent and the world devoid of divinity, for a new scientific, hyper-rationalist age where there's a potential to return to an understanding of the world as sacred with the support of data from sophisticated levels of quantum physics and neurobiology. She expands on this theory, saying, "The dominant culture is still characterized by capitalism and autocracy, where the world we live in has no sacred component – it's inanimate and we're at the top of the pyramid. We're at a moment of reckoning. It could certainly get worse before it gets better. So how do we return to right relationship? For me, that's a relationship that experiences the world in which we live in the full measure of its mystery as sacred. We begin to attend to it as a spiritual teacher, as a practical guide that can show us how to live in a sacred way, as part of the sacred world. Not as the ruler or dominators, but as a strand of this tapestry of creation, with a moral and aesthetic role to play."

As we sit in this transformational moment, our experts suggest we can learn lessons from our ancestors to shape how we move into the future. I must say, I was a little sceptical about this when I first heard the idea from Phyllis Curott, but having sat with it for a while, it starts to make sense to me.

She says, "When I ask the spirit of the place wherever I am anywhere in the world, 'What do you need?' one of the first requests that I get is always joy. I think a message from the past from when we were in right relationship with the Earth was that the offering of our joy to the world evokes a response of joy from the world. That's the message for all of us to remember from our past relationship with the Earth, that was always a liminal space, we were in this sacred relationship where the divine could show itself to us, and we could see it and that evoked in us joy, and our relations with the Earth were joyful. That's what we need to remember of our past, before we move into the future. That wisdom from the past is there for us. It's a blessing that carries forward that we have to learn again. Open and let go of the bad parts of our past, and this memory comes forward, this ancestral memory of joy and gratitude. That creates the future."

The wisdom that Bruce Parry takes from his time living in tribal communities around the world with regard to our relationship with nature and the planet is multifaceted. In addition to the importance and power of community and shared values, he talks about their healing modalities and medicines that allow for the release of emotional and mental health issues and an understanding of them, "rather than the prescriptive way we have of just taking a pill to avoid," as he puts it. Largely, what he takes is a sense of meaning and belonging that you get from living in a community. He says, "Knowing who you are, knowing where you're from, knowing the place, knowing the ancestors of there, having a belief in the spirit realm and a connection with the environment is something that you get. Also knowing your impact on the environment because you see it, it's much more local. We don't of course, because we export it over the hill, and only now it's coming home to roost. We find it really hard to undo that because we've become so accustomed to the luxuries and privileges that we have."

From Surviving to Thriving

It seems to me that part of being in the liminal is trusting and waiting until the right answers come. In the case of the planet, much damage has already been done and many of the practices that cause the greatest damage are under scrutiny while we decide what actions to take next. Yet, how do we know what the Earth needs?

To Phyllis Curott, the answer is obvious. We get out into the natural world and allow nature to make her magic, and if we pay attention, we will get the answers. She says, "We're smart enough monkeys to be able to figure out what we need to fix, and then we have to fix it. Then we go to the next step. And the next step is kind of natural – it's that feeling of gratitude and the reverence that follows, and the desire to give back when you recognize how much you've been given – life itself. You move from a survival motivation, which is what's going on right now, to thriving. And to thrive, then we have to be in harmony. So, then, you start paying attention and you start to see that natural laws actually reflect deep spiritual wisdom.

"It's a process. You don't unmake 5,000 years of false consciousness in five minutes, but we only have about five minutes. So, we all have to do the very best we can. We have to be patient with ourselves and support one another as we make better and better choices. We each have to do a little bit; this every day can add up to big changes, especially if we all do our small part. We just have to be realistic about how dangerous the moment is and optimistic about our capacity to make the changes that can fix what is broken and what is dangerous."

While Parry is condemning of our institutional response to the COVID pandemic, F**k It philosophy founder John Parkin is looking for the silver lining. He says, "We've seen for probably the first time in our lives that, at times, the state really needs to step in. We've been brought up in a neoliberalistic economic view. What's happened with the pandemic, given it's been a massive emergency like a war, the state has come in and gone, 'This is what you guys need to do. This is what we all need to do, and you're going to pay more for this eventually. You'll have to pay more taxes.' And I'm hoping that that was a great rehearsal for what we'll have to do with climate change. Governments will go, 'Well, we got to have a go with COVID. We didn't do it trans-globally and we didn't do it together, but what we did is we all stepped in, you all followed what we had to do, you realized it was important that we operate at the state level. Now we have to do the same thing for the environment, because we're all dying.' So, I'm hoping that will happen."

What seems clear to me is that our stay in the uncertain space between a previously abundant and generous world and, depending on the choices we make, either a world beyond redemption or a salvaged world is coming to an end. Our sojourn in the liminal is over and a decision one way or another is needed.

The one consoling thought is that the natural world has amazing regenerative and restorative capabilities. As Sadhguru points out, "As human beings, we cannot escape anything that happens to the planet because what you would call 'myself' is just a piece of this planet. Did you know if human beings disappear from this planet, trees will break through concrete and grow through houses? Everything will thrive wonderfully. They say if the insect population in the world dies completely tomorrow, within 25 years, all life on this planet will end. But if you and I vanish, everything will flourish. That is a clear statement as to where we stand in this world."

I shall give the last word to the inspirational Earth wisdom of Phyllis Curott, who concludes, "What gives me hope is the innate capacity of the Earth to heal and the power of rebirth. If we just stop inflicting harm, she recovers much more rapidly than we thought possible. Chernobyl is going to remain toxic to humans for millennia but there are wolves now in Chernobyl, because their lifespans are short enough that they're not affected by the radioactivity. Fascinating, right? So, if we simply stop abusing the planet, then we have to start contributing to the healing – net zero is not enough. We have to remedy, we have to do good, we have to make things better. Yet, if we simply cease, then she has this power of regeneration, of rebirth, of healing, which is extraordinary.

"Long-term, the planet will reset and restore itself. Short-term, the loss of any living species because of our neglect, greed, stupidity and fear is a tragedy that could throw you into a prolonged depression. But, we're useless like that. I made my commitment to do my small part and to do the best that I can in the time that I have here, to help people get the blindfold off and rediscover that they are living in a sacred world, which is showing them how to live in practical ways that are also sacred. In fact, there is a moral compass operating with all of this. Everything is contributing to the overall wellbeing of the planet and the wellbeing of all of us. That's the way we're supposed to live. That's how we're supposed to create social, economic, political and commercial institutions, by asking ourselves, 'Is what we're doing making the world a better place?' Not just zero emissions – that's a very low standard. No, ask ourselves, 'Are we contributing to making this world more welcoming for all life, not just human beings, for all life?' That's the moral creed."

Liminal Life Lessons

It may at times feel like any actions that we take toward a greener lifestyle are just a drop in the ocean compared to the remedial actions required from governments and industry. Nonetheless, each small contribution helps and the gathering momentum of individuals joining pressure groups, supporting green political parties and becoming eco-activists is creating a movement that is almost impossible for the powers-that-be to ignore.

Essentially, the overall message appears to be that we should be realistic about the danger that we find ourselves in at these liminal crossroads, and optimistic about our capacity to get this right.

Here are some of the personal actions that our own group of experts is implementing and their advice for activities that we can consider or adopt.

Expert Inspiration #One

Satish Kumar believes that, "We have been exploiting nature and exploiting people. We have to give back. What can we give back? Our time, our talent, our skills, our craft – making things. So, the giving and receiving, the principle of mutuality and reciprocity, should be brought back into our everyday life. Without mutuality, without reciprocity, without receiving and giving to one another, hand in hand, there is no quality of life."

Expert Inspiration #Two

The best action recommended by Sadhguru is that we all become more politically active. He says, "Only when governments are elected on the basis of promises they make to correct ecological damage will there be a real solution. We are putting across this idea of a 'Conscious Planet' movement. There are 5.2 billion people living in countries with the ability to vote and elect their nation's leadership. We are looking to get three billion people on board so that ecological issues become the issues that elect governments. We want to make them aware of at least five ecological aspects that must happen in their country, and two or three aspects that must not happen. If we do this, then ecology will become if not the number one, at least the number two issue in election manifestos."

Expert Inspiration #Three

Here are some of the practices that Phyllis Curott has adopted in her own life and that she suggests to others. She says, "We all have things that we can do. We have shifted to not an entirely vegan diet, but a much more vegetable-based diet. It's one thing that everybody can do that makes a big difference. I don't buy new clothes because clothing is one of the most destructive misuses of resources and generators of pollution on the planet. It's not just about choosing organic and cotton, because in fact cotton uses a lot of water and does a lot of damage. So, most of my clothes are used. Figure out something that you can reduce, recycle or reuse. You know, I put on layers and reduce the temperature of the thermostat in our house. And I'll keep it low. Ask yourself, 'what are the things that we can do to reduce our footprint?' The people whose job it is to analyse this have told us, if we can drop our own footprint by about 15%, that would have a huge global impact – just enormous. You have to pick energy companies that seem to be making the right choices and moving in the right direction. You have to vote for the right people. All of us have to be far more engaged in politics than we want to be because we are looking at a global wave of authoritarianism.

"Our job, as spiritual activists, is to think clearly, listen attentively, share what nature shows us, be courageous. Pick the changes that we'll make in our daily lives and then pick the thing to which we'll commit ourselves in activism. Periodically, I get scared to death and deeply worried. Then I come outside and make my offering. I feel the deepest gratitude and in feeling that deep, deep gratitude, I'm allowing the beauty and the dynamic energy of nature to inform my soul and my mind and my body to get into harmony. And I remember where I am. In remembering where I am, I remember why I'm here. And that's to help do my little piece to fix what we've broken, and I get to work."

My Chapter Take-aways

- Before we can change our relationship with nature or adopt a reverential ecological approach, we have to be more comfortable in nature, more familiar with it. We can each start that reconnection just by getting outdoors more often and by being present and observant when in the natural world. Walking barefoot on the grass is a good place to start if this is all new to you, and then expand your horizons from there.
- There are some great initiatives across the planet, albeit that more are needed. Do you feel moved to join a local group or to get involved with an eco-activist movement? If not now, then when?
- It feels as though we have hovered in this liminal space on the brink of ecological disaster for so long that it's hard not to be discouraged or disengaged. Yet, my position is that I remain hopeful that there is still time to avert a global catastrophe. Despite the enormity of the challenge, I continue to recycle, to litter pick and to eat as cleanly as possible. A drop in the ocean possibly, but for me, it dilutes my feelings of insignificance and impotence.

FINAL THOUGHTS

Thank you for joining me on this journey of enquiry through liminal space. There's a lot here to digest and consider, and I hope you have found it interesting. Perhaps you will feel stirred to explore the liminal, in all its guises, in your own life more.

Although I've enjoyed sharing my thoughts on liminality with you, and those of the experts, I've realized that sometimes how you feel about something does not need explanation. The liminal has a noetic quality that defies explanation.

I still feel drawn to seek out liminal spaces and thin places, to take pilgrimages through the landscape to sacred sites and to go on solitary walks in nature. My love for these spaces has been enhanced by what I have found out during the researching of this book, but I suspect I would still love them without any knowledge to substantiate my passion. Similarly, I continue to reap the benefits of being taken off to another place during my meditation practice, and now know a little more about why it's helpful and what I'm tapping into.

So, what other nuggets of wisdom have I picked up along the way? I believe that some of our deepest self-knowledge is revealed to us in the pauses in our lives and the natural transitions that are visited on us. Our greatest inspirations and inventions are discovered in times of uncertainty. For me, the vast unexplored territories on the edge realms of our consciousness hold more allure than the edges of our cosmos, and just as much mystery. Holding communion with something greater than ourselves, a higher power, can only be achieved when we surrender ourselves to the liminal, when we put our trust in something unattestable.

Ultimately, it seems to me that knowledge and certainty are slippery customers. Although we have a natural distrust of change and a love of homeostasis, we are also curious by nature. It is in asking the questions, of ourselves and others, that we gain a greater insight into the deeper meanings of life. Sitting with the question, feeling our way into the answers, being okay with the not knowing for sure, is how we get a sense of who we are and how we fit into this world, and a better understanding of how we wish to live our lives going forward. There are distinct benefits to learning to love the spaces in between.

ABOUT THE EXPERTS

One of the delights of writing this book was the willingness of the contributors to give freely of their valuable time and knowledge in interviews with me. All showed such enthusiasm and passion for their aspect of liminality, and their combined wisdom is awe-inspiring. Here is a brief introduction to each of them.

Dr Eben Alexander had over 25 years' experience as an academic neurosurgeon in Boston when, in 2008, he was driven into a coma by a rare bacterial meningo-encephalitis. He spent a week in a coma on a ventilator, his prospects for survival diminishing rapidly. To everyone's surprise, he woke after seven days with memories of a fantastic odyssey into another liminal realm. Ever since, he has brought key insights from his journey to the mind-body discussion and our human understanding of the fundamental nature of reality with his books, including *Proof of Heaven*. I was lucky enough to hear of his experiences direct from the horse's mouth and I can say without hesitation that Dr Alexander is one of the most erudite and inspiring people I have ever interviewed.
ebenalexander.com

Having worked in publishing for years – as a non-fiction editor for Simon & Schuster and Head of Publishing at Gleam Titles – **Abigail Bergstrom** threw her life up in the

air and herself into the liminal when she left her job and her home in the middle of the pandemic. As such, she is no stranger to the possibilities that lie within the liminal. She has now started her own publishing consultancy, Bergstrom Studio. When I read about what she had done in *Vogue* magazine, I knew I had to interview her for the book and I was delighted when she agreed.
bergstromstudio.co.uk

Yasmin Boland is a moonchild who teaches about the Moon, the Divine Feminine and astrology. A former journalist and TV producer turned astrologer and bestselling author, Yasmin has been working with the Moon and scouring the skies for insights for nearly 20 years. Who else do you turn to when you want a discussion about lunar cycles?
yasminboland.com

Michael Boyle was one of the first people who sprang to mind when it came to the chapter that included rites of passage. His most recent project Breaking the Spell is specifically designed to support men and women to liberate themselves from restricting personal and cultural conditioning. But it was his work as the Founder of Abandofbrothers, a charity providing rites of passage experiences and male mentors for local disaffected young men, that I knew would be of great value to this book. He didn't disappoint.
abandofbrothers.org.uk   *mankindproject.org*

I simply love talking with **Phyllis Curott**. Who better to chat to about the power of the liminal within the natural world – a subject close to her heart? An attorney, writer and one of America's first public witches, Phyllis' bestselling books, and her YouTube series *What is Wicca?* with over 2,000,000 views, have introduced the world to witchcraft. She is the founder of the Temple of Ara, America's first and oldest shamanic Wiccan tradition, and is the first Wiccan Trustee and Vice Chair Emerita of the Parliament of the World's Religions. After a hiatus from the public limelight and an apprenticeship with Mother Earth, she has returned to writing and lecturing internationally on the embodied spiritual wisdom of Mother Earth, nature's 'secret magic' and why the world needs its witches.
phylliscurott.com

Alison Davies is a regular contributor to *Kindred Spirit* magazine and I knew her extensive knowledge of storytelling and natural cycles would be invaluable to this book. As well as running workshops at universities, Alison also has a keen interest in folklore, health and wellbeing, and the esoteric. She's a great believer in the power of storytelling as a tool to enhance communication and deliver a powerful message.

New York Times bestselling author **Dr Mike Dow** has a Doctorate (Psy.D.) in Psychology and also a post-doctoral education in neurofeedback, psychopharmacology, bilateral-based therapy for the treatment of trauma, and clinical hypnosis. As the American media's go-to expert on brain health, he is immensely busy, so I was hugely grateful when he made time at short notice to talk to me about the liminal space we enter when in an altered consciousness. He could not have been more gracious, enthusiastic or interesting.

drmikedow.com

Danu Forest is a traditional wisewoman in the Celtic Bean Feasa tradition of her Irish ancestors, seer, druid witch and priestess, with 30 years' experience studying the Celtic mysteries. Noted for her quality research and practical experience as well as her deep love of the land, I know her best as a regular feature writer for *Kindred Spirit*. She is the author of several books including *Wild Magic*, *The Druid Shaman*, *Celtic Tree Magic*, *Gwyn ap Nudd* and *The Magical Year*, and she was the first person I thought of for the chapter on the opportunities for growth offered by the liminal spaces of the seasonal cycles in the natural world. Danu is just so knowledgeable and wise – I couldn't have asked for a better contributor.

danuforest.co.uk

One of the pioneers in the revival of the women's wisdom traditions, **Eliana Harvey** is the founder of Shamanka, a unique school of women's shamanism. She has been involved in the spiritual path since 1960 and, when I met her, I felt like an initiate at the feet of the great teacher – she simply has a wealth of wisdom that she shares with such joy and willingness.

shamanka.com

Dr Robert Holden's innovative work on psychology and spirituality has been featured on *The Oprah Winfrey Show, Good Morning America* and in two major BBC documentaries called *The Happiness Formula* and *How to Be Happy*, shown to over 30 million television viewers worldwide. He is the Director of The Happiness Project and Success Intelligence, and he hosts a weekly radio show called *Shift Happens!* He is also the author of the bestselling books *Happiness Now!, Authentic Success* (formerly titled *Success Intelligence*), *Be Happy, Shift Happens!* and *Loveability*. Phew! And yet he happily made time to talk to me at length about destination addiction.

robertholden.com

I never tire of talking with the wonderful **Glennie Kindred** – we have so many common interests. She is an artist and a writer, with twelve books currently published, the latest being *Walking with Trees*, all of which include her artwork. Her books explore the wild edges of our relationship with the Earth through our native plants and trees, tree lore, herbalism, Earth wisdom, alchemy, celebrating the Earth's cycles and creating heartfelt ceremony. She is also the editor and co-creator of the yearly publication, the *Earth Pathways* diary.

glenniekindred.co.uk

Peace-pilgrim, activist and former monk **Satish Kumar** has been inspiring global change for over 50 years. Satish was the editor of *Resurgence & Ecologist* magazine for 43 years and now serves as Editor-emeritus of this much-loved publication. Satish also co-founded Schumacher College in South Devon and continues to teach and run workshops on reverential ecology, holistic education and voluntary simplicity. He is a much sought-after international speaker. I'm so pleased he made time to talk to me about reverential ecology and his experiences as a pilgrim, providing another valuable perspective.
resurgence.org/satish-kumar

Maggie La Tourelle is a writer, holistic therapist and teacher, based in London and Findhorn, Scotland. In her therapy practice Maggie integrates counselling, psychotherapy, NLP coaching, kinesiology and energy work to bring about health and wellbeing in mind, body and spirit. Her ground-breaking work with dementia care is available in workshops and seminars, and in her book, *The Gift of Alzheimer's*.
maggielatourelle.com

I found talking to **Samantha Lee Treasure** fascinating. She became interested in the anthropology of Out of Body Experiences (OBEs) after her own recurring experiences in 2009. Alongside her studies, her aim is now to offer helpful information and answers to experiencers and the general public in an ethical, neutral and unbiased way. It brought a smile to my face

when I saw that Samantha lists liminal spaces and states as one of her interests on her website – something we have in common.
zombiesinpjs.com

I have met **Denise Linn** several times over the years, and was lucky enough to attend one of her workshops. She is remarkable. Denise is an internationally renowned teacher in the field of self-development. She's the author of the bestseller *Sacred Space* and the award-winning *Feng Shui for the Soul*. Founder of the Linn Academy, Denise created and taught certification programmes in life coaching, Feng Shui, space clearing, clutter clearing, oracle card reading, dream coaching and much more. Hearing about her experience of and wisdom in running visions quests was invaluable to me and to this book.
deniselinnseminars.com

Caroline Myss is a five-time *New York Times* bestselling author and internationally renowned speaker in the fields of human consciousness, spirituality and mysticism, health, energy medicine, and the science of medical intuition. Caroline established her own educational institute in 2003, CMED (Caroline Myss Education), and she maintains a rigorous international workshop and lecture schedule all over the world.

In 2020, Caroline released a book on prayer, including 100 of her personal prayers, *Intimate Conversations with the Divine*. I love this book – it sits on my bedside table and I dip into it frequently. You can imagine how delighted I was when Caroline agreed to an interview – a rare privilege – about the liminal nature of belief and the power of sacred language.

myss.com

Maestro shaman **Chris Odle** trained in the Mestizo shamanic tradition in Peru in 2004. Since then, he has been running La Medicina plant sanctuary in the high jungle of the Peruvian Amazon. It was a pleasure talking to him about ayahuasca ceremonies and the traditions of the indigenous people.

I couldn't have been more pleased when **David Olliff**, a regular feature writer and columnist for *Kindred Spirit* magazine, agreed to be interviewed for the chapter on divinity. With a first-class honours degree in Theology and a keen, enquiring mind, I felt sure he would have a valuable contribution to make. He didn't disappoint.

John Parkin is the author of the bestselling 'F**k It' books, and, back in 2008, I attended one of his F**k It retreats which he and his wife Gaia run in various spectacular locations (such as on the volcano of Stromboli) in Italy and the UK. We subsequently became friends and I wouldn't have wanted to write this book without including his insightful and original contributions.

thefuckitlife.com

Bruce Parry is a filmmaker, award-winning documentarian, author, indigenous rights advocate, explorer, trek leader and former Royal Marines officer. I was so delighted when Bruce agreed to be interviewed. His film, *Tawai: A Voice from the Forest* is powerful and moving. When my sons were small, we would watch his BBC documentary series *Tribe* and his ayahuasca experience stayed with me – hence the call. *bruceparry.com*

I have interviewed **Anthony Peake** before, and I always come away feeling slightly dazed by the sheer breadth of his knowledge. This time was no different. Tony has now written eight books – all develop his 'Cheating the Ferryman' hypothesis about consciousness into ever-wider areas of application. His latest book is *Cheating the Ferryman: The revolutionary science of life after death*. *anthonypeake.com*

A philosopher and author, **Daniel Pinchbeck** is perhaps best known for his online magazine, *Reality Sandwich*. His other published works include *How Soon is Now?* and *Breaking Open the Head: A psychedelic journey into the heart of contemporary shamanism*. In *When Plants Dream*, co-authored with anthropologist Sophia Rokhlin, he looks at the global spread of ayahuasca and it was great that he was able to talk to me about that aspect of his work together with his views on altered consciousness. *pinchbeck.io*

Author **Victoria Preston** and I roamed the moors above my house while I picked her brains at length about the importance and value of pilgrimage. Her book *We Are Pilgrims* shows us that journeys of meaning and purpose are always a powerful reminder that we are each part of something much greater than ourselves. I highly recommend it.

Born Jagadish "Jaggi" Vasudev, **Sadhguru** has been teaching yoga in southern India since 1982. In 1992, he established the Isha Foundation. Sadhguru is the author of several books and a frequent speaker at international forums. His latest initiative is the Conscious Planet movement, focussing on ecological issues.
isha.sadhguru.org

As a nurse in a British hospital for 21 years, 17 of those in intensive care, **Penny Sartori** was ideally placed to conduct unique and extensive research into the Near Death Experiences (NDEs) of her patients. I was delighted when she agreed to share her thoughts and research findings with me, which I found fascinating.
drpennysartori.com

Steve Taylor is a senior lecturer in psychology at Leeds Beckett University, and the author of several bestselling books on psychology and spirituality. His new book

is *Extraordinary Awakenings: When trauma leads to transformation*, which of course piqued my curiosity for this book. In fact, I have met up with Steve Taylor before for interviews and his research is always breaking new ground. Eckhart Tolle has described his work as "an important contribution to the shift in consciousness which is happening on our planet at present."
stevenmtaylor.com

I have followed **Felicity Warner**'s work for many years, ever since we first met at a literary lunch in the early noughties. She published her first book *Gentle Dying* in 2008, and created the idea of Soul Midwifery for the dying after sitting with many hundreds of people at the end of life. Her pioneering work over the last twenty-five years has brought a new dimension to holistic and spiritual palliative care, both in the UK and abroad. She is a respected lecturer, teacher and author of four acclaimed books, one of which, *The Soul Midwives' Handbook*, is a textbook used by complementary therapists and in medical and nursing schools.
soulmidwives.co.uk

I loved hearing in his own words the story of **Neale Donald Walsch**'s now famous Conversations with God experiences. The series of books that emerged from those encounters has been translated into 37 languages, touching millions and inspiring important changes in their day-to-day lives. Neale's views on the divine were a valuable addition to the book and the question of what the liminal space is we inhabit when we commune with divinity.

nealedonaldwalsch.com

FURTHER READING

Bergstrom, A, 2021. Inbetweeners. *Elle magazine.*

Boland, Y, 2016. *Moonology: Working with the Magic of Lunar Cycles.* London: Hay House UK Ltd

de Botton, A, 2014. *The Art of Travel.* London: Penguin.

Campbell, J, 1949. *The Hero with a Thousand Faces.* Princeton: Princeton University Press.

Gennep, A, 1969. *Rites of Passage.* New York: Johnson Reprint.

Holden, R, 2022. *Higher Purpose.* Carlsbad: Hay House Inc.

Kindred, G, 2013. *Letting in the Wild Edges.* East Meon: Permanent Publications.

Kindred, G, 2011. *Earth Wisdom.* London: Hay House.

Moran, B, 2016. Wake the F**K Up. London: Watkins Publishing.

Myss, C, 2021. *Intimate Conversations with the Divine.* Carlsbad: Hay House Inc.

Parkin, J, 2022. *Fuck It: The Ultimate Spiritual Way.* London: Hay House UK Ltd.

Peake, A, 2022. *Cheating The Ferryman.* London: Arcturus Publishing Ltd.

Peake, A, 2006. *Is There Life After Death?* London: Chartwell Books.

Pinchbeck, D, 2014. *Notes From The Edge Times.* New York: Jeremy P Tarcher.

Resurgence & Ecologist, magazine.

Ring, Dr K, *Life At Death, 1980.* New York: William Morrow & Co.

Ring, Dr K, *Lessons From the Light*, 2006. Moment Point Press.

Sartori, P, 2017. *Transformative Powers of Near Death Experiences*. Readhowyouwant.

Sutton, N, 2021. *Consciousness Rising. Carlsabad:* Hay House Inc.

Walsch, N, 1997. *Conversations with God [New ed.]*. New York: Hodder and Stoughton.

Walsch, N, 2020. *The God Solution: The Power of Pure Love*. Phoenix Books Inc.

ACKNOWLEDGEMENTS

It is such a pleasure to be able to publicly thank and show gratitude to all those who supported me through the at times challenging process of writing this book. A big thank you to those who believed in it, even when I was unsure – Jean, Jane, Lizzie – and for the unstinting support of my husband Nick and my two sons, Alex and George. I'm grateful too for the wonderful professional expertise and backing that I've received from Chelsey Fox, my agent and friend, and the amazing folk at Welbeck – Jo Lal, Kate Latham and Beth Bishop. Thank you all.

Finally, I would like to thank the inspiring experts who enthusiastically gave up their time to talk to me about liminal space. Their contribution cannot be praised enough and I am truly grateful.

ABOUT US

Welbeck Balance publishes books dedicated to changing lives.
Our mission is to deliver life-enhancing books to help improve
your wellbeing so that you can live your life with greater clarity
and meaning, wherever you are on life's journey. Our Trigger
books are specifically devoted to opening up conversations
about mental health and wellbeing.

Welbeck Balance and Trigger are part of the Welbeck
Publishing Group – a globally recognized independent publisher.
Welbeck are renowned for our innovative ideas, production
values and developing long-lasting content.
Our books have been translated into over 30 languages in
more than 60 countries around the world.

If you love books, then join the club and sign up
to our newsletter for exclusive offers, extracts, author
interviews and more information.

www.welbeckpublishing.com   **www.triggerhub.org**

🐦 welbeckpublish   🐦 Triggercalm
📷 welbeckpublish   📷 Triggercalm
📘 welbeckuk   📘 Triggercalm

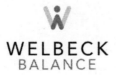

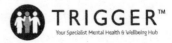